# live well
# with louise

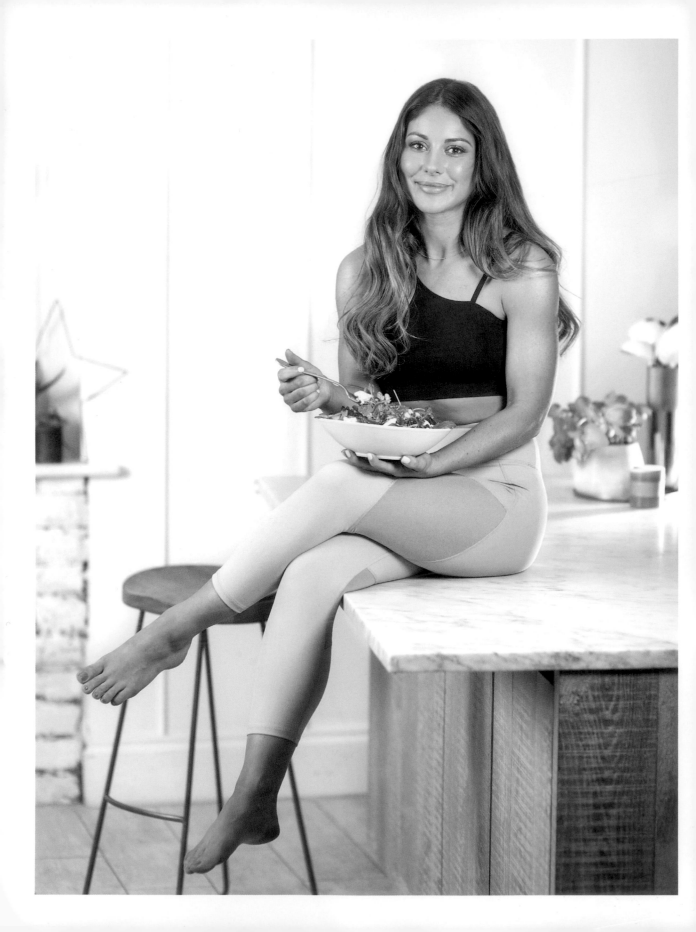

# live well with louise

## fitness and food to feel strong and happy

### LOUISE THOMPSON

PHOTOGRAPHY BY ANDREW BURTON

First published in Great Britain in 2018 by Yellow Kite
An imprint of Hodder & Stoughton
An Hachette UK company

1

Trade Paperback ISBN 978 1 473 67735 7
eBook ISBN 978 1 473 67736 4

Editor: Lauren Whelan
Project Editor: Laura Herring
Design and art direction: Nikki Dupin
Photography: Andrew Burton
Prop styling: Olivia Wardle
Recipe development / writing and food styling: Kat Mead
Nutritionist: Kerry Torrens
Personal trainer: Ryan Libbey

Colour origination by BORN
Printed and bound in Italy by L.E.G.O. S.P.A.

Hodder & Stoughton policy is to use papers that are natural, renewable and recyclable products and made from wood grown in sustainable forests. The logging and manufacturing processes are expected to conform to the environmental regulations of the country of origin.

Yellow Kite
Hodder & Stoughton Ltd
Carmelite House
50 Victoria Embankment
London
EC4Y 0DZ

www.yellowkitebooks.co.uk
www.hodder.co.uk

# contents

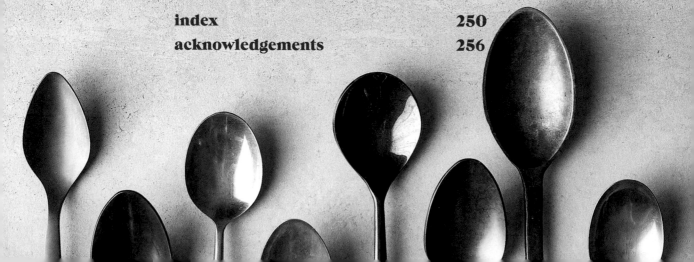

# my journey

I always thought that writing an autobiographical book at a young age was a little arrogant and self-righteous – what does anyone at this stage of their life have to tell the world? The old me used to be a lot more judgemental. I'm now a firm believer that if you have something to say that might benefit others then you should speak up about it...

Up until this point, details of the personal journey I've been on to find a happier, more optimistic place have been kept under wraps. I haven't even spoken to my parents about what I've been through and most of my friends only know part of the story, because – despite being in the spotlight on one of the UK's most popular reality TV shows for the last seven years – I'm a fairly private person. Opening up publicly is a huge deal for me, but I know now is as good a time as any... I've spent much of my twenties battling anxiety, struggling with confidence and feeling quite unhappy for the most part, I just wanted someone to tell me that everything was going to be OK. The last couple of years have been a game changer and my biggest realisation is that I do have the power and tools to make positive changes to my frame of mind; we all do.

My main aim with this book is to reach out to readers who might relate to my struggles and to some of the decisions I've made in the past, and hopefully show them that there are ways to move forward and improve your outlook for the future. Changing up your daily routine may make a massive difference, in the same way it has for me. Although it has been a big, fat, steep learning curve, I'm now clear about the things that make me feel better and the things that make me feel worse. Discovering new activities and passions you enjoy has the potential to lift the cloud and reignite your spark; for me it was food and fitness – so this is where the focus of the book will lie.

Between the ages of 18 and 25 I think it's safe to say I was in a dark, confused state, despite having it all 'under control' on the surface. I used to bulldoze through, never stopping to deal with my emotions, I wasn't kind to my body and would end up repeating the same self-destructive cycles until I reached rock bottom. This may not seem particularly unusual for a twenty-something, but when you're neglecting your mental and physical health for a sustained period in favour of late nights, a poor diet and minimal movement; it will take its toll and deplete your energy. I wish I had made a few fundamental changes to my lifestyle sooner as this would have saved me a lot of stress and self-loathing. My life was exciting for sure and I don't regret all the things that happened during this time – I had fun, but I lost myself along the way and was left empty and directionless. I lived *for* the moment, not *in* the moment and had no idea what made me happy anymore. A sense of impending doom and panic became the norm so I accepted it and embraced it as best I could.

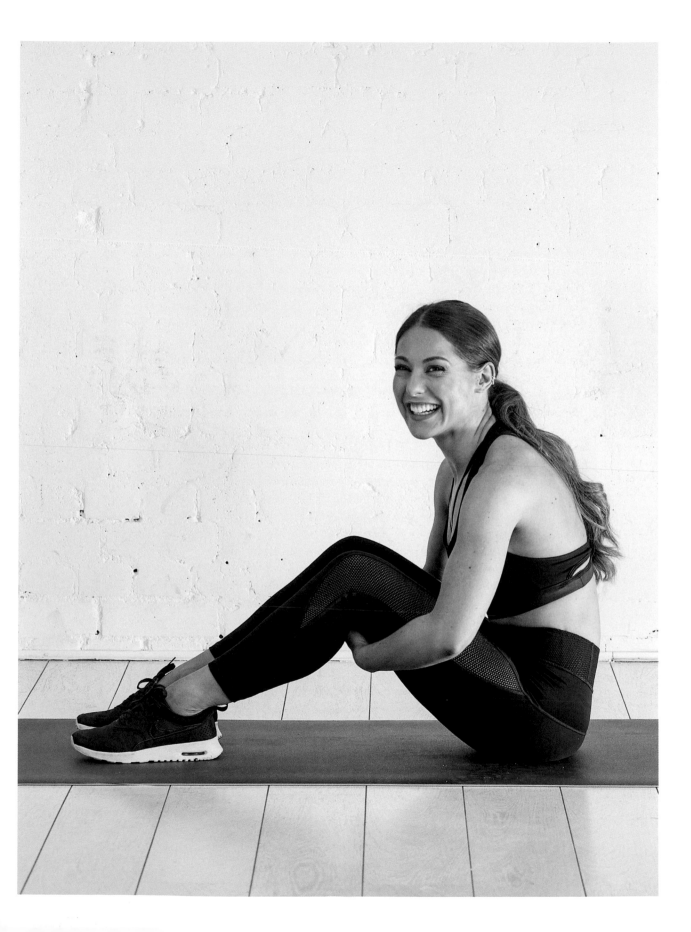

I am the first to admit that I have made plenty of mistakes. You know how people say that you shouldn't have regrets because you learn from them and it shapes who you are? For me that statement is arguable, but I have learnt to accept the past for what it is instead of letting it consume me with worry and fear. After all, the mistakes have led me to where I am today. It is all part of growing up, working out what is truly important and what makes us happy. The reality is, when we're lacking in confidence and not looking after ourselves it can lead us to make questionable decisions that can send us into a downward spiral. My downward spiral cost me a lot of friends, money and memories. But I managed to get myself out of it, repair my outlook, cut out the negativity and turn things around slowly, but surely (it just took some commitment!). I am now much stronger, mentally and physically, and as a result I am able to make better, more confident choices for the future.

 **I am now much stronger, mentally and physically, and as a result am able to make better, more confident choices.**

Having intimate details of your life and relationships broadcast for the world to see (tears and all!) can leave you feeling vulnerable. I will never complain about the opportunities that I've been lucky enough to have because of my public profile, but it hasn't always been rainbows and butterflies. I've been subjected to a great deal of online abuse in the past, which has been tremendously hurtful. During complicated patches in my personal life, the negativity would roll in thick and fast. However, I now receive thousands of messages from people who take time out of their days to write to me and tell me how much better, stronger, happier, fitter (the list goes on) I seem to be, and who want to know my 'secret' and what changes I made. I want to thank every single one of those people because without this positivity and support, I wouldn't have been inspired to write this book. When I am a target for negativity these days, I am less affected by it; I know that other people's comments are out of my control and having a better sense of who I am as a person makes it a hell of a lot easier to block out the haters. I've learnt to take everything with a pinch of salt and to try to be grateful for the good things in life. It is important that you don't let other people's opinions define who you are and where you're heading. Remember that social media is not a reflection of real life.

Changing how I eat and exercise has been a major factor in my growth in confidence and renewed direction; these outlets allowed me to reroute and start fresh with zero expectation when I felt my lowest. Regular exercise has had an incredible effect on my mental health; it eases my anxiety, slows my racing mind and boosts my mood when I'm overwhelmed and on edge. It has taught me to trust myself and my ability, and given me the space to just breath, when all else fails. I can't wait to share my favourite home workouts as this is something I have had a LOT of requests for. I'm even sharing my secret ab blast routine... Minimal equipment, no expensive gym membership needed; you can do them anywhere at any time of day. I wanted to make them as accessible and doable as possible!

I used to resort to working out and yo-yo dieting as a short term fix to distract myself from life's stresses or in a desperate attempt to lose weight. I developed a destructive relationship with both and overlooked how much joy they could bring me. Committing to being active and fuelling my body with fresh home-cooked food is now vital to my day. They hold the key to a positive, calmer me. One of the sections I'm the most proud of in this book is my recipes which I hope you'll enjoy making too. I've never professed to be an amazing chef, but I've completely fallen in love with cooking. The ritualistic nature of getting creative in the kitchen and experimenting with delicious new flavours (even when it is a super simple thrown together dish) brings me so much pleasure and comfort! Like exercise, the simple, physical act can help us to relax, switch off and focus on the present moment.

I can't deny that the process of being honest has been cathartic, and I'm grateful to have had the opportunity to put pen to paper for the first time. It's important that we try to stay on the right path once we have found it and celebrate the simple stuff in life that makes us feel good. We all veer off track, we just have to keep going and remember to be kind to ourselves. I don't beat myself up about a missed workout or over-indulgence, and nor should you. Of course, I have days where I'm struggling to see the positive – who doesn't? – I will share with you how I focus my mind during these times and offer up my tips on how to stay motivated. I hope that my journey will inspire you to make the changes you want to make or encourage you to open up and find someone to talk to, whether that is a close friend or your GP; there is help out there if you need it. We're a generation that is finally taking mental health seriously and sharing really is caring. For me, a happier wellbeing is about getting stronger in every sense; eating good food, being active, a walk in the fresh air, discovering activities you enjoy, connecting with people, embracing imperfection and letting go of the past. Big things start small and gradual improvements to your outlook will be worth it in the long run, we are all a work in progress!

Let me know how you get on! #LiveWellWithLouise

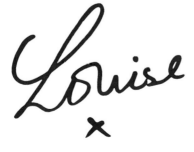

x

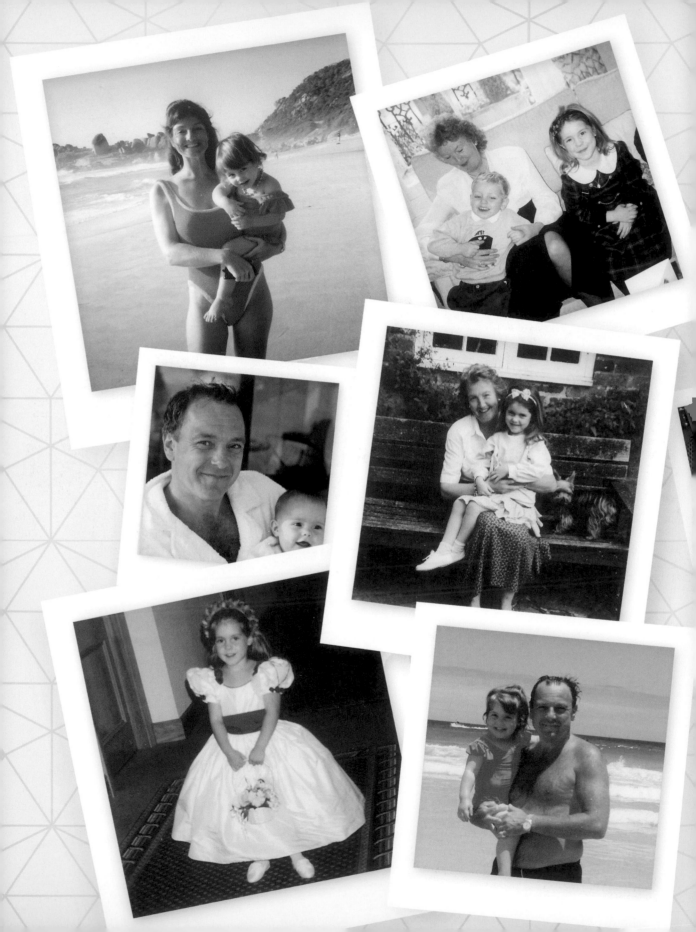

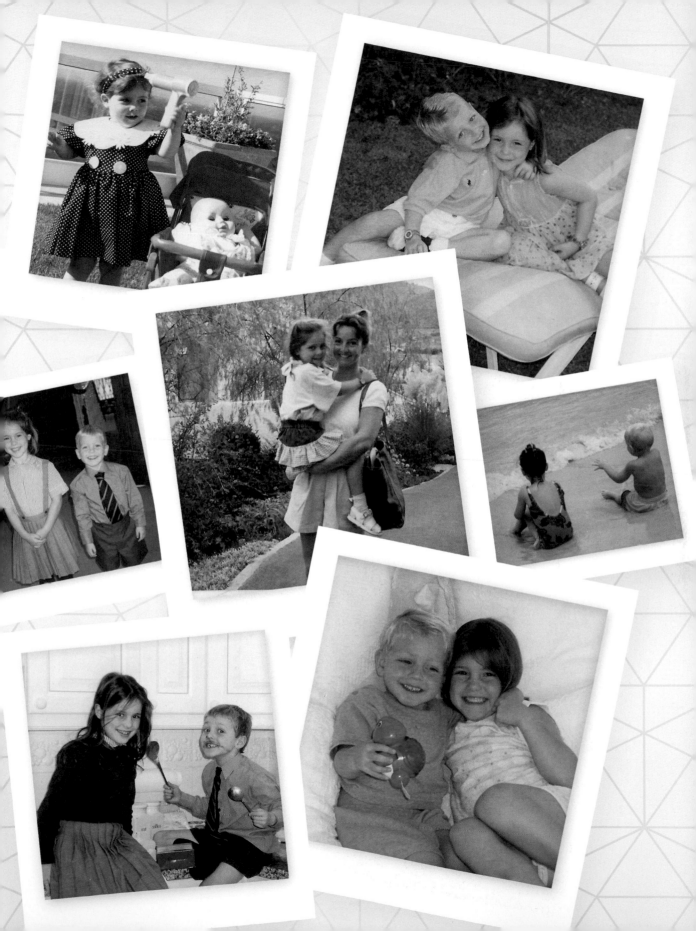

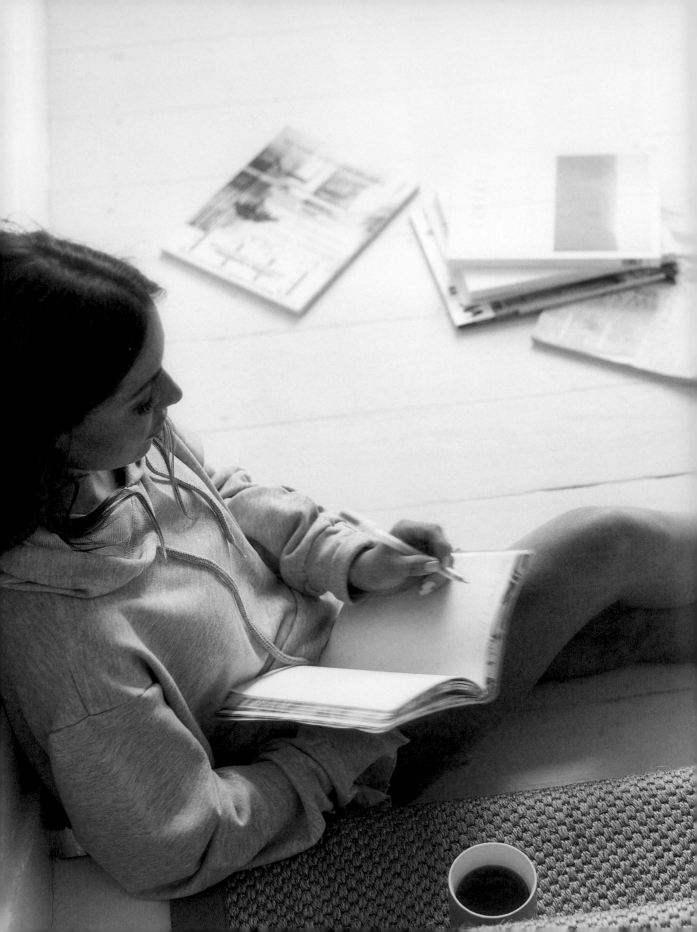

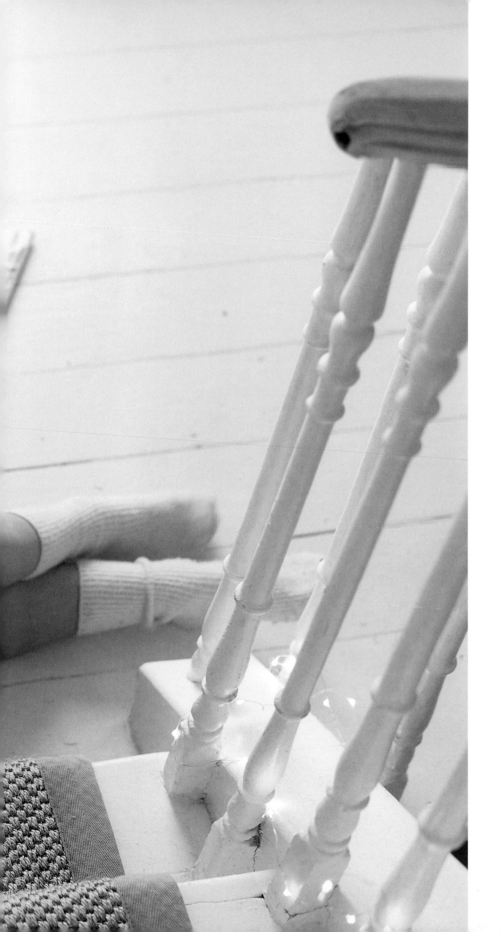

something
had to change

PART 1

# a bit about me...

We can all look back with the benefit of hindsight, and try to work out where and why certain behaviours and habits started. Although it's impossible to tell whether we would be the same people we are today (for better or for worse) had we done things differently, when I look back over my life so far I can definitely see where some of my feelings of insecurity began.

Like most of the population, I was never skinny or long-limbed. In fact as a schoolgirl, I was stocky and always a lot shorter than every other girl in my class. I am asked about my height ALL THE TIME, so now I can put a stop to the speculation, I am bang on 5ft. I am aware that this is under average, but it honestly didn't bother me back then. I was lucky to come from a happy, loving home, and went to boarding school when I was 11. I found it surprisingly easy to adapt to being away from home, probably because I have always been good at being told what to do! But I put a lot of pressure on myself to do well and I struggled to engage with the things I found difficult. I would get very upset, often resorting to crying when I couldn't do things as well as I wanted to, even when I hadn't put in enough work.

As far as food went, I ate three large meals a day, with plenty of traditional school puddings. We played competitive sport at least three times a week, which meant we burnt it all off, and no one ever considered what 'healthy eating' even was. No social media meant there were less constant comparisons with other people online, and no 'healthy' bloggers or skinny models to follow. The only comparable outlets that we were exposed to were fashion and gossip magazines. Ignorance was bliss.

The moment I left school it became immediately clear that I had no idea how to live without being instructed on what to do all the time. I suppose, on reflection, that was when I started to become uncertain about who I really was – although I don't expect this is an uncommon way to feel at that age. I took a job to earn money to travel before university, and combined 5am work starts with a lot of partying and late nights. I started dating someone who worked in a nightclub, and hanging out with a whole new set of people. We had a wild time, but I became flaky with my family and old friends, letting them down regularly. I went from being well-behaved to flying off the rails in order to fit in with my new friends. I even got fired from my job which was quite a low point .

Then came my degree. I remember being in Brazil and spending many hours in a very slow internet cafe checking to see whether my various uni applications had been accepted. It was

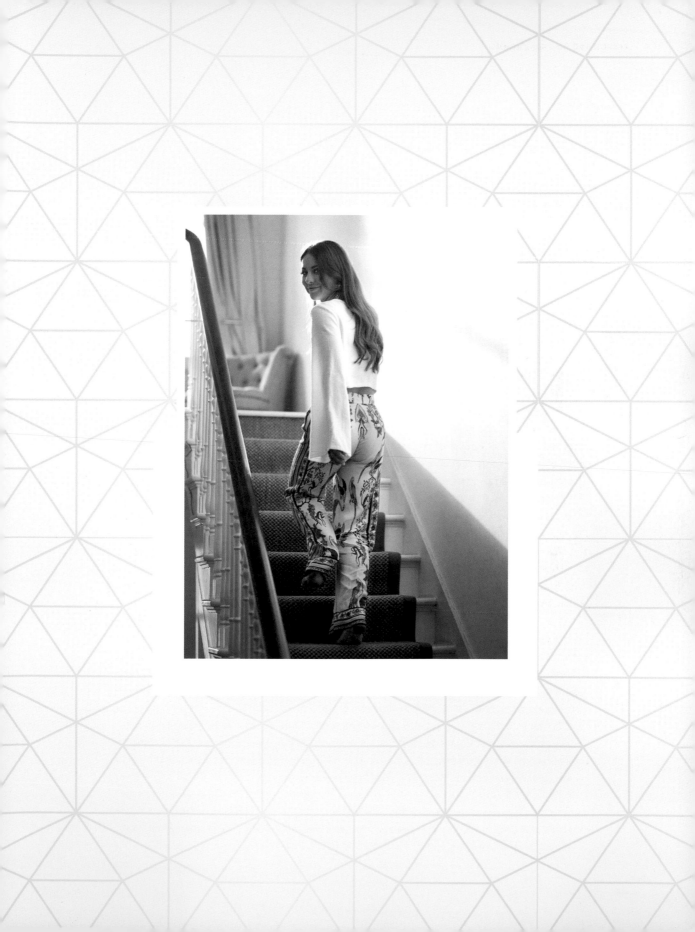

incredibly nerve-racking because Edinburgh (my first choice) was the last university to process their applications and announce their decision. When I finally found out the good news that I had been accepted I was thrilled that all my revision and the slightly avant-garde personal statement I'd written had paid off. It amuses me to cast my mind back to the moment I was asked to make a choice on what I was going to study and where I wanted to go because at 18 I was pretty naive and I hadn't done a lot of my own research. We had 'careers' lessons at school, where we were given options of jobs we might be suited to, but most people ended up following the crowd. I think the real reason I decided to study so far away was simply because Edinburgh had a reputation for having a brilliant geography department. I had visited the city during the summer for the Fringe Festival and I loved it, plus I already knew I could handle being far from home from being at boarding school so young. However, I didn't realise when I started there that I would soon take on a job in London that would change my life.

## made in chelsea

I hadn't planned to join the show and sort of fell into it because I find it difficult to say no. The producers were keen for me to join midway through the first series because I had friendships with the existing cast. After several phone calls back and forth, their relentlessness paid off and I said I would try it for a one-off scene, this then snowballed into me becoming one of the main characters. In this instance, I'm incredibly lucky that I am such a 'yes' person because it has led me to where I am today.

I'm ashamed to admit now that I'd been quite rude about *Made in Chelsea* when it first came out – I thought it was a bit low-brow and a waste of a good education. But now I can admit I owe a lot to it. It has created opportunities for me, and we also won a BAFTA, which was a pivotal moment in television so I'm delighted to be a part of that! But it hasn't been easy working in an environment where you are opening your entire life up to the criticism of the general public, and I often found myself revealing more than I planned to on screen. My feelings towards the show have evolved with each series; sometimes positive, sometimes negative; there are definitely some moments I'm not proud of... The stress of filming while studying for a degree, along with having a social life often felt too much. I was probably the most honest person in the cast, and that left me really hurt and vulnerable at times. A vicious cycle developed where the more hurt I was, the more it seemed that people hated watching me, and the nastier they were online. People are very quick to make judgements, and I was on the receiving end of some horrible comments. There have been several occasions where I trended worldwide on Twitter, but it was never for any favourable reasons. It turns out that people would much rather comment on the bad than the good, and they will say things online that they would never say to your face. Since then I've learnt that it is only a very sad type of person who would take it upon themselves to waste their time bullying others online whilst pathetically hiding behind a keyboard. My lowest point was around five years ago when, NO EXAGGERATION, I would receive hundreds of negative comments every second over the course of an hour on a Monday evening. There were thousands in total. I remember in my final year at uni I would sit in my room and check my phone to get a grasp of what was happening in the episode because I didn't want to watch it with my flatmates in the living room, mainly out of fear of embarrassment. Strangely, I've only ever been able to watch the show with people who work on it, probably because we share a mutual understanding of the way it is created.

That level of negative feedback is inconceivable to me now. I do still find it hard to get my head around how much people care about what I do, but back then it was far more prevalent. I signed up for a television show, so I have to accept the fact that viewers are going to have an opinion, but bullying is never acceptable. I felt as though people totally misinterpreted my behaviour and I had zero control over this. Many of the comments were slating my appearance and comparing me to various animals, which is hard to take in your early twenties. How I look has no relevance to the content of what is shown on TV; considering it is not a beauty pageant. In addition, I would be threatened with strict advice on how I should live my life from complete strangers. People said I deserved to get cheated on. And then there were the death threats from a select few. Death threats are ILLEGAL.

I once recognised someone who had been trolling me online at an appearance I made during a university freshers' week; she was incredibly friendly to my face and even asked for a picture together. I didn't call her out, instead I let it slide, but it was proof that I shouldn't listen to the fickle judgement of people who don't even know me – often people will criticise for the sake of it. This isn't only restricted to the realms of social media.

At first I had no idea how to battle the negativity; I soon realised there was little point in deleting the comments because there were simply too many of them. Responding to them would only lead to satisfaction on their part, so I chose to just ignore it all. Choosing not to rise to it was definitely the right move, but I think deep down my ego was torn to shreds. I'm happy that people are starting to recognise that negative behaviour online is not OK and users are now regularly being called out for their damaging trolling activities.

Nowadays, I receive a lot of sympathetic or supportive comments and positive questions, especially since I've been in a better place. Of course, I welcome the questions and I try to respond to people because I am a very social person and I love the interaction, but I think it is good not to get too affected by comments online in terms of how it makes you feel about yourself. It can have a harmful effect on a person's confidence and ego at either end of the spectrum. Don't let social media and other's opinions define you.

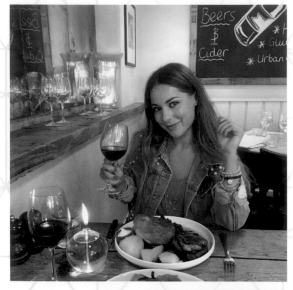

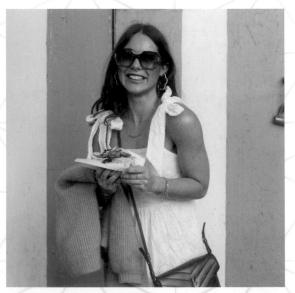

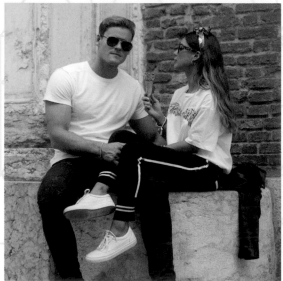

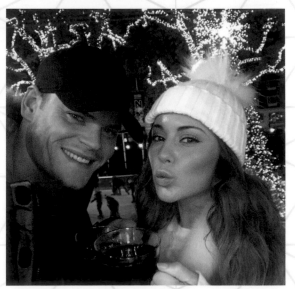

# unhealthy choices

While I was trying to balance filming and studying, my diet and lifestyle suffered hugely from the lack of any proper routine. I would often turn up to filming without having had a sufficient lunch and stuff myself senseless with anything I could find in the snack box, which was typically chocolate, crisps and sweets. Then I'd think, 'Oh well, I've already eaten quite a lot so I might as well just write this day off and binge until I feel sick or finish a whole large packet of something'. This was my life most days of the week. I would have 'healthy eating' or detox days in between to make myself feel less guilty.

My 'healthy eating' would typically involve cutting out all carbohydrates. That was the only diet I knew, but now I know that without a certain amount of complex carbohydrates and a balanced diet I'm not going to be able to achieve what I want, or look and feel how I want. Instead, I will be depleted of energy and utterly miserable. Eating properly is important for my health, to feel good, and to maintain my weight. When I would 'detox' I would drastically reduce my calorie intake to an unhealthy level; in essence, I was yo-yo dieting. But most of the time I was eating whatever was in sight because that was my way of dealing with the pressures of studying and filming at the same time. I felt sorry for myself and would compensate with a LOT of treats and comfort eating, occasionally polishing off two large pizzas at a time.

I also developed a really unhealthy relationship with alcohol. Drinking too much started for me when I was with my first ever boyfriend – who cheated on me twice. We dated in my late teens when I was very impressionable. Although I forgave him and we got back together, the trust was knocked. That was around the time I also started comparing myself to other girls too. I got myself into a horrible cycle of thinking that I was never good enough and so I would drink to feel better and more confident. I saw it as a way of coping with my issues with self-esteem, and I would do four times a week what most people did once in a blue moon, to blow off steam. I would get so drunk that I found it hard to remember what had happened the night before and this became a habit I continued all through the years to come.

While I was drinking like this, I made some questionable decisions that didn't just make my life difficult, but ended up hurting other people. I would constantly wake up the next day racked with guilt and worry from my mistakes, as well as feeling that I was throwing away my education and everything else I'd been given. This constant low-level anxiety on top of an excruciating hangover meant I would spend around three days every week full of panic and self-loathing while trying to pick up the pieces from the mess I'd created. It was a vicious and destructive cycle that I was inflicting on myself.

# Being healthy isn't about the weight you lose, it's about the life you gain...

My relationship with drinking cost me not just friendships, but most of the money I was earning. I lost over 30 phones, five handbags and had my car towed 25 times because I couldn't make it the next morning to move it from where I had parked it. I wasn't a bad person, but I was a people pleaser. I basically had a big problem saying NO and it was clear to me, in my sober moments, that I was spiralling out of control fast; losing any sense of normality and who I was as a person.

My personal relationships were also complicated around this time and I definitely had issues with love and dependency. I jumped from one relationship straight into the next, becoming completely involved with that person and then feeling depressed when it ended, even though deep down I knew they weren't right for me. I would push them to the point of having no choice but to break up with me by acting irrationally and then beg for them back because I couldn't bear being on my own. While I did love being on *Made in Chelsea* and would never change my decision to join the show, I found myself envying my friends who had much simpler lives than mine. I questioned whether I had experienced too much too young and what direction I was really headed in. I was lost and in quite a bad place mentally.

For FAR too long I knew I needed to make big changes, but I didn't know what they were or how to implement them. The longer it went on, the more overwhelming it seemed: where was I supposed to start? In my late teens and early twenties, I think everyone, including my friends and family, assumed that I had my life pretty sorted. After all, I had been lucky enough to have had a secure, loving upbringing and a supportive family I could rely on. But behind the façade, I knew that I was struggling to cope with the way I lived my life. Of course, I now know you can't just sit around waiting for a magic wand to make everything better, which seems obvious – but when you are lucky enough to grow up in the relative privilege that I did, it can take a bit more figuring out.

After years of living on this rollercoaster, feeling insecure and fundamentally unhappy, I knew that things couldn't go on the way that they were. I wanted clarity. I craved a healthier, happier, and calmer lifestyle. Things came to a head when I woke up one day in bed at my dad's house after going to a club the night before. I felt so physically unwell, to the point at which I thought I was dying – either through anxiety or through severe dehydration, but probably a mixture of both. I knew then that the first step to feeling better was to start properly looking after myself. I had stopped treating my body with the respect it deserved and it finally caught up with me.

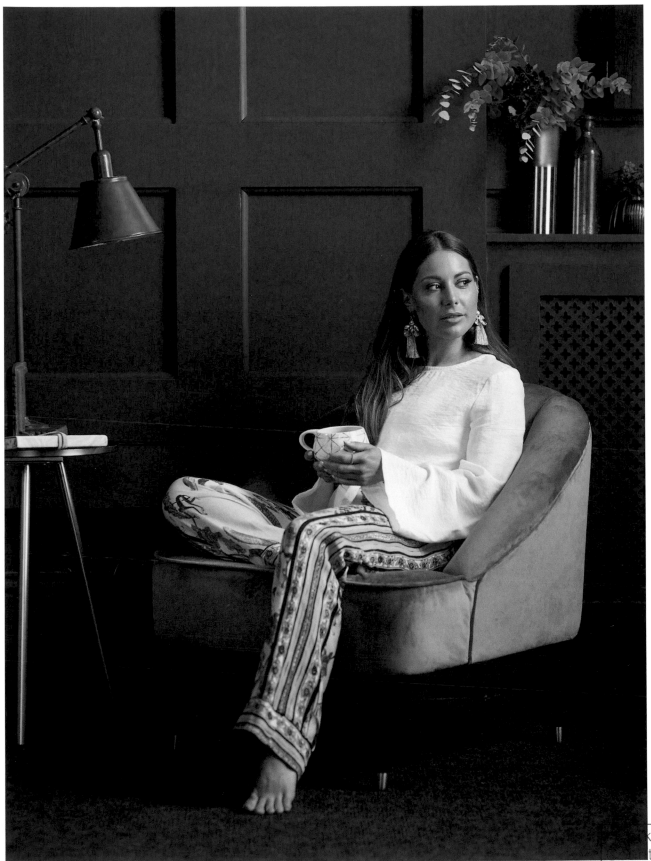

# first things first

I had reached the stage where I needed to sort out my life and take charge of my mental and physical health. I hadn't felt properly myself for some time and I was tired of my present existence. I had been planning to move to New York with a boyfriend, but I kept making excuses for not moving because I was too cowardly to admit the truth that we shouldn't be together, and that moving Stateside wouldn't fix much deeper-rooted problems. I knew I had to find the courage to end the relationship and do what was best for ME. When I finally did, I felt such a sense of empowerment. Having been instructed on what to do at school for years and then to a certain extent been directed by the TV show, it was a huge relief to break the boundaries and start working out what I wanted – to strip my life back to basics, get stronger on my own, and to finally start prioritising myself over pleasing others.

## say NO…

In order to start fresh I had to make some sacrifices and to learn how to say no, which had always been a problem for me. This was the first and probably most important step. I stopped saying 'yes' to every invitation. This was beneficial to both myself and the host because I wasn't running myself into the ground with excessive socialising and I wouldn't have to call up hungover to bail on the invitation an hour before the party, letting people down. I cut my social diary to 10 per cent of what it used to be and it was a huge relief. My mother always told me that I needed to stop agreeing to everything, but it took me 25 years to finally accept it. I have NO idea why I ever agreed to do so much in the first place. Since committing to far fewer things I seem to have much more fun when I do go out. I only do things that I'm actually going to benefit from and enjoy. I never benefited in any way from all those blackout drinking nights because I wasn't even creating any memories, I was making myself feel worse. The only people who created memories were those around me reminding me how stupid I had been on a night out, which left me in a 'humiliated' and paranoid state for days after.

That brings me to my next point.

# eliminating toxic relationships

Unfortunately, in life, there are some people who will sabotage your self-improvement. Often they aren't even aware they are doing it, so it isn't their fault. But this is about you, not them. The word toxic is very strong but what I mean by this is anyone who does the following:

- **Someone who tries to control you.** Anyone who tries to manipulate you often isn't in control of their own life.

- **Someone who influences you to make bad decisions.** Toxic people thrive off of making your life as messy as theirs.

- **Someone who doesn't take responsibility for their own actions.**

- **Someone who is negative.** People who always see the cup as half empty and those who complain all the time. I used to be a bit like this and now I make a conscious effort not to be – after all, positivity breeds positivity.

- **Someone who is judgemental.** This is the WORST sort of person to surround yourself with. There are a few people I used to hang out with that I couldn't be myself in front of. You should always be yourself around your friends.

- **Someone who takes more than they give.** The issue of give vs. take is unlikely to ever be in perfect harmony, but if someone brings no value to the relationship then it can be frustrating. For example, friends who unload on you when they're going through a rough time, but aren't there for you when you need them.

- **Someone who tells you that you can't.** Be a lone ranger if you have to in order to achieve your goals and dreams.

You have to accept that distancing yourself might be a gradual process. Lots of people are threatened by the idea of change. I used to be this way inclined, but I made the decision to change my life quite considerably, so it was important I wasn't surrounded by people who didn't want similar things.

I didn't do anything dramatic to get rid of toxic influences. It wasn't necessary to owe anyone an explanation or apology or block them on social media. I didn't send a letter or meet face-to-face. To be honest if I'd met up face-to-face I would probably have ended up being sucked back in. Instead I gradually distanced myself from those people. I think this was easy(ish) for me at this stage in my life because in your late twenties everyone seems to go in their separate directions. All my good friends are more settled now and working hard towards their futures. People don't go out and get wrecked as much. There is still a group of people who do go out every night to distract themselves from their day-to-day lives, and I avoid this group like the plague. Because that is what I used to be a part of. It's interesting when I look back to that time in my life and realise that I felt most lonely when I was in that group, permanently socialising and surrounded by people.

I've learnt that I used to be toxic too.

## eat better

Your body and brain will thank and reward you almost immediately for this. Your diet lays a firm foundation for how you feel. I started spending time cooking at home, fuelling my body with good nutrition and I felt far happier and more energised almost at once. By good nutrition, I mean healthy eating. And by healthy eating I don't mean following a diet, I mean including all food groups and not depriving yourself of anything.

I replaced some refined grains with whole grains, for example, eating brown rice instead of white rice. I tried to eat less sugar and salt. I threw a few extra helpings of fruit and vegetables into my food preparation. I avoided greasy takeaways and ready meals, except on the very odd occasion. I cut out the junk food and started creating meals from scratch every night. I packed healthy snacks like fruit and nuts to take to filming so I didn't binge on chocolate bars. I also massively cut back on the drinking. I would never totally abstain from anything because I think this puts too much pressure on me, so I still have the odd glass of wine with dinner or a glass of champagne if I'm out celebrating – but I no longer go out with the sole aim of getting drunk and I don't get out of control. Within a few weeks of making these changes I saw a huge difference, not only physically, but also to my mental health. With a well-fuelled body, I have more energy and am better equipped to deal with the everyday stresses that life throws at me.

## exercise regularly

It's hard to feel bad about a body you take care of. I had to make changes by setting goals and having a vision for what I wanted to achieve. I knew in the past that when I'd exercised it made me feel good, so I thought if I was committed to making it a REGULAR occurrence (instead of a quick fix) then it would improve my overall wellbeing. I decided that my goal was to do some form of exercise at least three times a week. At the beginning this might have only been for 30 minutes a session, but for me this was the optimum amount that I could achieve whilst staying on top of my work and getting adequate sleep and allocating some 'me time' too. After a few weeks, I felt happier, brighter, and more in control of my life. It gave me a space to slow down, switch off and breathe. As a by-product I noticed that I built muscle and stamina too, which encouraged me to keep going. Even simple tasks like running up and down the stairs became easier. I felt mentally and physically invigorated every time I left the gym. I started living my whole life at a faster pace, and became more efficient in my daily life again. The cloud over my head started to lift...

At first I was motivated by joining classes. One of my new aims was to be less wasteful with money; if I booked them in I knew I couldn't bear to lose the money so I would have to go even if I couldn't be bothered. I tried a lot of different classes until I found the ones that I liked and was good at, with the best teachers. I know classes can be pricey, but if you shop around there are some great deals. I think it is really important to have variety in your workouts, so you shouldn't be afraid to try new things. I started tracking my progress by writing down my workouts and I would take screenshots of the distances I'd done on any machines I used. I would also take pictures in a sports bra and shorts to see how my body gained strength.

I used to hate fitness, but – maybe because I started doing it for the right reasons and not purely for the aesthetic value – I have fallen madly in love with it. First and foremost, fitness is about the positive effects it has on my mindset. It encourages me to embrace what I'm born with and trust myself. Eventually I found the confidence to try exercises using weights, such as shoulder presses and weighted squats, moves I'd previously associated with big, burly men. I was instantly hooked! I found a passion for something and I was good at it. I realised I didn't need to break into a sweat to totally transform my body composition. The benefits inspired me so much that I kept at it until exercise became an irreplaceable part of my life. I had discovered an outlet and focus that I enjoyed.

I suppose I was lucky that Ryan fell into my life at the right time, when I became passionate about training, and of course he has helped me along the way. He taught me how to perfect my technique and has encouraged me to keep pushing myself. But it is in no way essential to date a personal trainer to get awesome results! Once you know the fundamentals, you can start your own journey. And there will always be people willing to help.

## leave the past behind

You can't start the next chapter of your life if you keep re-reading the last one. I had to teach myself this in order to move on. I used to obsess over how I could have done things differently. I would beg and beg for forgiveness, and for someone to change their mind about not wanting to be with me, but you have to accept that everything happens for a reason, and some things are not meant to be. This applies to all aspects of your life. Sometimes my past still bothers me because I feel like I've wasted so much time making mistakes. But more than that I resent the fact that I've wasted time worrying about everything! There is nothing you can do to change what has already happened. The best thing you can do is learn from it and not repeat the same mistakes. These days I find it helpful to reflect on how far I've come, but I don't dwell heavily on the past as I know this leads me to a place of unnecessary anxiety.

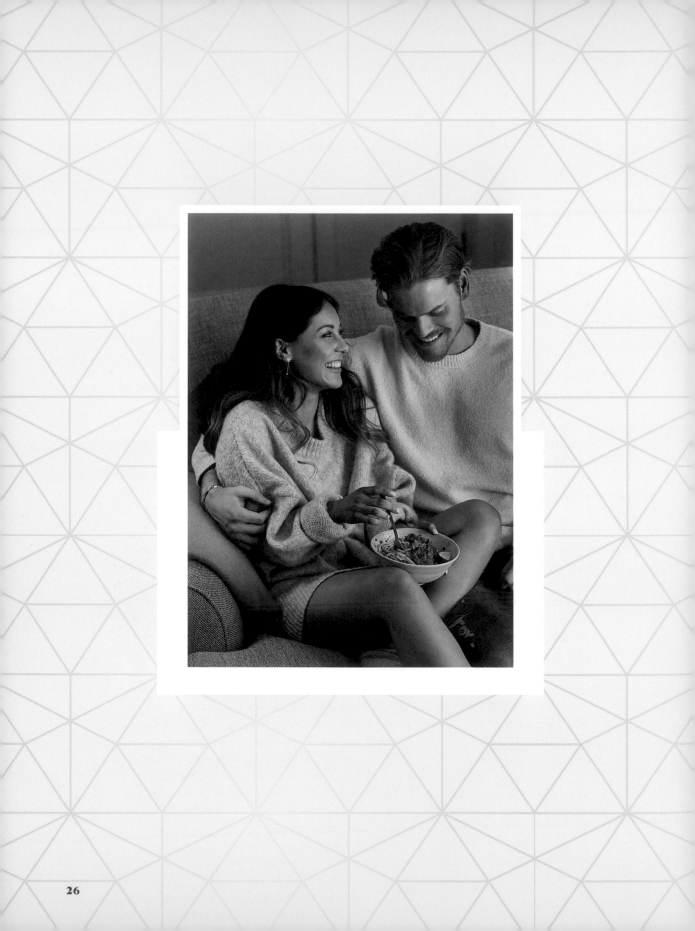

# keep checking in with yourself

To make sure I'm staying on track, I ask myself a series of questions. Asking questions can be tough because we don't want to have to confront our thoughts. However, I believe that progress can't be made without pushing yourself into an uncomfortable zone and recognising how you're actually feeling. Of course, there are no right or wrong answers.

**My list of questions I ask myself to make sure I stay where I want to be:**

- Am I doing the things I know I should be doing in order to feel good?
- What did I learn today?
- What do I want my life to be like in five years?
- Make sure I give back – who or how did I help today?
- What am I grateful for?
- Am I having enough fun?
- What is my Number 1 priority right now?

I find these kinds of questions really determine the life that I lead. When I read them they trigger emotions and answers which then influence how I act and behave on a daily basis. If you aren't happy with your answers then start making some changes. For example, if I have a day where I don't feel like I've learnt anything then I will make sure that I try to do a totally random and spontaneous activity the next day. It doesn't need to be anything crazy, it can be as simple as having a conversation with someone you wouldn't usually talk to. Last weekend, for instance, I went to Columbia Road flower market in London to do some research and learn a bit about gardening. The more I listened, the more I learnt. I'm also a total nerd and like doing online quizzes, testing myself on new things, such as capital cities, US states, historical events etc. The internet is a never-ending source of knowledge and inspiration.

I love the question, '*What are you grateful for?*'. I went through a phase of forcing Ryan and myself to say something we were grateful for before going to bed each night. This might be excessive but every now and then you can write it down on some paper somewhere and then it's nice to look back and read through it. There will always be something to be grateful for, even if it's having your health, or good food to eat. Get rid of anything that doesn't fill you with positivity. Finding my positive place has totally changed my outlook on life.

# feeling stronger

I might be five feet small, but I am powerful, and that for me is the best thing I've achieved. I love the fact that women are getting to redefine femininity by opting for a much broader choice of body shape that goes way beyond the supermodel waif-life ideal. It means that we can value our bodies for what they can do rather than just how they look, and that gives us all a different, more inspiring yet totally realistic ideal to achieve. When you are physically strong and have developed that faith and trust in your own body, you naturally become more confident and mentally strong too.

We are all imperfect in our own wonderful way. Perfection doesn't exist, however much the media feed us a perceived idea of it. I've been on TV for seven years and received all sorts of comments about the way I look. Whether it's ego-boosting compliments or soul-destroying insults, none of it is acceptable or helpful, as I talked about earlier. How we perceive ourselves is a delicate subject. I realise that in other people's eyes I've never been exactly out of shape, but that doesn't mean I was happy, or that it was wrong to want to change the way I approached fitness and body image in general. Whatever size or shape you are, it's not for anyone else to tell you what you can or can't change about yourself. Nor to make you feel compelled to change something you are OK with just to look like everyone else around you. There is only one you and it's up to you how you choose to portray yourself to the outside world.

I developed a full-blown complex about my arms at the age of 14 after a negative comment from someone and for about 10 years I didn't wear anything that revealed them – I thought they were bulky and masculine. For the first few years of filming *Made in Chelsea* I would wear a jacket any time I was required to wear a sleeveless dress, even if it was somewhere boiling hot, which would result in sweating profusely, but that's how desperately distorted my body image was. Through exercise, my arms haven't got thinner – in fact they're probably just as muscly, if not more – but I now don't see any problem with revealing them. I don't care what anyone else's arms are like, or what anyone thinks of mine; I love the fact that they are strong and I couldn't be prouder of them!

I had also developed an inferiority complex over being short because everyone on television seems to be a glamorous 5ft 10. I've always been teased for being 'vertically challenged', and people would constantly ask me how tall I am. When I would watch an argument that I'd had on the TV I immediately felt like I had a disadvantage because of being looked down on. There was something so patronising about it. I've been spoken to in baby voices a lot, because people think I'm 'cute'. I was infantilised by people, especially men, who underestimated my intelligence, strength and ability.

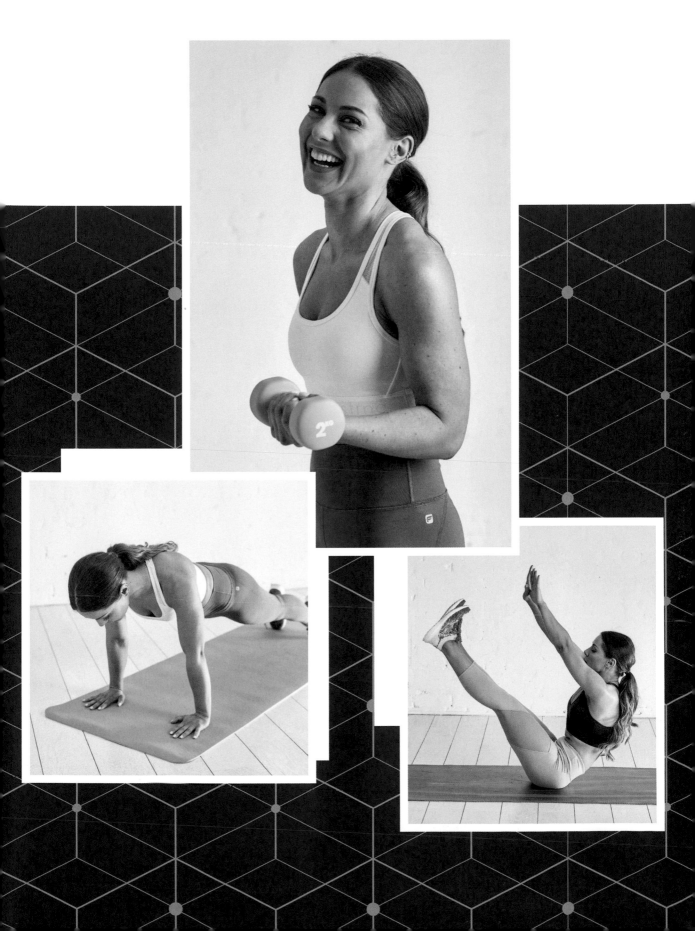

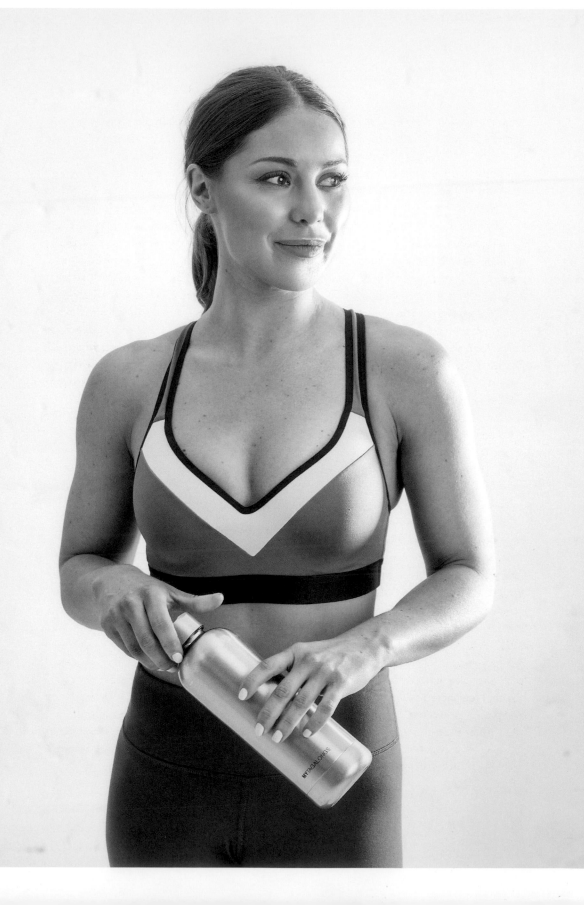

The first step is to **STOP COMPARING YOURSELF TO ANYONE ELSE.** As soon as I accepted who I was and that I couldn't change the length of my limbs, or my genetics for that matter, I became instantly happier. In the age of social media overload, avoiding comparisons with others is harder than ever, but it is important to remember that people mostly only post their best moments, and that it isn't a reflection of real life. I know the game as I have a large following myself and I can't deny Instagram has given me a powerful platform, BUT I'm fully aware that most people only post the best of everything because I'm guilty of it too. I don't go around posting pictures of me and my boyfriend when we have a huge argument or when I have cystic acne on my chin, or when I'm lounging around the house in my Disney pyjamas. It's only the BEST selfie, the most TONED abs, the FULLEST hair shots that are shared for the world to see. I'm sure the intention of social sites is as somewhere to post what you enjoy doing and the things that reflect you and your world, but it's crucial to put these images in perspective and not let them make you feel negative about yourself. Take a step back when it is no longer making you feel good. I am grateful that Instagram wasn't a thing when I went through my most devastating break-ups, as I know the younger version of myself would have wasted hours stalking my ex's new flames – social media can just fuel the fire of that unhealthy habit of comparing yourself to others.

There has also been such a historic trend to critically scrutinise the way we look. We have been bred with a lack of ability to compliment ourselves, or even accept compliments from others. I once turned around to my friend's mother who told me I looked good and said 'F*** off, I don't,' because I was awkward about receiving a compliment. Things got even more awkward after that... Learn how to absorb the loveliness of a compliment.

Being too critical of yourself can lead to a road of negativity, despair and an unhealthy dose of self-consciousness that can leave you feeling miserable. Over the past few years I have developed a more forgiving attitude towards my body. I don't weigh myself because I don't want to become obsessive over anything. We need to learn to do what feels right for our body. Not everyone can follow the same routine, or eat the same food. Stop trying to be perfect. The place I personally want to be is one where I love the way I am, but am still encouraged to make some positive changes; there are always things that can be improved. We are all born with different bodies, and it's up to us what we do with them. I've played to my strengths, and although some people might think my figure is too muscly and turning boyish, I feel incredible. I'm not going to change for anyone, and I'll certainly never please everyone. I've learnt to try and live a happy life, in my own way, and if I can sprinkle even just one reader's day with a little bit of the positivity I've learnt to channel then that's amazing! I've come to see that being pint-sized isn't a problem, and what I lack in height I make up for in my determination to be a successful, strong woman.

# my battles
# with anxiety

Society has finally started to normalise the word 'anxiety' and it is being discussed in an open way. Feeling anxious or suffering with other mental health issues is something that many of us will experience at some stage of our lives (25 per cent, apparently). It is important to realise: 1) that you're not alone – sharing is caring; 2) it can creep up and surprise you at any time and often has no rhyme or reason; 3) you're just as entitled as the next person to feel what you're feeling (whether you're a man, woman, rich, poor, young, old) and 4) you will find things that can help and learn to avoid things that really don't – it might just take some time to work these out.

I've always been quite panicky – it's part of my personality. I grind my teeth at night, and even getting onto an aeroplane is a major struggle (don't even get me started on take off...). For a long time I've suffered with panic attacks. I remember a particularly bad one at university that lasted a few hours. I even experienced something called derealisation, which is a feeling of being totally disconnected from the world as if it isn't real. After this I didn't speak for ages because I was too scared it would happen again. I have honestly found anxiety to be more debilitating than any physical injury I've ever sustained.

For me, anxiety feels like an intense onset of fear and panic that you can't properly describe to those around you, probably because it is so different for each individual. Often I feel dizzy or light-headed and slightly confused, and then sometimes it develops into a sense of NEEDING to get out of a place and sit in a room on my own until I can compose regular thoughts. One of the things that offers most relief is being able to talk to my close friends about it. You will find out that plenty of people have suffered with similar feelings and it is incredibly reassuring to know you're not alone. I count myself lucky to now have an open forum with those closest to me, where we can talk openly and not feel like we are just unloading on each other. Having a network of supportive people around you is so important. Whether it is your friend, or your local GP, don't be afraid to start a conversation if you need help.

While I was in Edinburgh at university, I was out of the loop with what was going on during filming between the other cast members, including my boyfriend at the time. I felt as though every time I came back to London, spending about 40 hours a week on a train, I would have to deal with some unpleasant drama. That became such a recurring pattern that I would then worry about the onset of anxiety itself. I was permanently scared that I was going to burst into tears, to the point where I would work myself up so much before filming that it became a natural reaction to cry every single time, even if nothing bad was happening. I was losing my confidence and becoming scared of social situations, including my lectures and tutorials. I didn't really have anyone I could talk to who could sympathise with what I was going through. I was never sure whether I was doing things right or wrong, and every time the show aired I would face awful criticism from the public and this was tough to handle.

I suffered with bad social anxiety too, which you may find ridiculous considering I spend a great deal of time in front of the camera. But that life chose me as opposed to the other way around. I was not born to be a performer, in fact quite the opposite, I was actually very shy and self-conscious as a child. All of my friends at school seemed to do drama for GCSE and A Level, but I couldn't even pluck up the courage to audition for the school play, so it wasn't an easy road to get to where I am now.

When I was a child, I used to be too scared to ask the waiter for an ice cream on holiday. My dad wouldn't do it for me as punishment, so I just went without whilst my brother would eat his ice cream in front of me. I hated public speaking and talking to groups of people at university, and when confronted with it I would usually skip the class because I would go bright red and speak INCREDIBLY quickly. I had terrible social phobia whereby I was uncontrollably fearful of being judged by others. I was always paranoid that people were angry with me or that they didn't like me. Honestly, it has taken me around five years to be truly comfortable in front of the cameras, but looking back I'm glad I never gave up because perseverance did pay off and I FINALLY got to where I want to be. Now I'm in a place where I love what I do and finally have a clear sense of who I am; on and off screen.

 **For me, anxiety feels like an intense onset of fear that you can't properly describe to those around you.**

I feel as though I have had a fairly loud life full of ups and downs, as each year unfolds into a different mini life. I am relatively experienced for a 28-year-old, and carry a fair bit of emotional history and baggage. As I've said, I don't regret the things that have shaped me, but it has been a rocky road and there have been some real lows. I hope that I have put my darkest periods behind me.

However, I think I will always be susceptible to feeling uneasy. Now I am better equipped to deal with social situations and have learnt how to look after myself, I seem to have developed a whole different breed of anxiety whereby I perpetually worry about my health. It's important for me to set myself some reminders in order to manage my negative thinking.

## my helpful reminders:

- It is important to be different, that's what gives you an identity.
- Mind your own business, don't worry about what others are doing.
- Choose wisely when it comes to what you care about.
- Be patient. Time is a great healer, and you are in control of your own destiny.
- Don't be so narcissistic, the chances are people aren't even thinking about you.
- Stop seeking approval through other people, have faith in yourself.
- Stop making mountains out of molehills. Move onto something constructive.

I've learnt that sometimes you have to put yourself first, especially when it comes to your mental health. As mentioned earlier, a big step for me was getting rid of negative influences, whether that was relationships or friendships, and I stopped putting myself in difficult situations that I knew would affect me badly. As I changed my way of thinking, things got a lot better, slowly but surely.

A major factor has been focusing on treating my body with respect, eating a balanced diet, and clearing my mind so I can focus on what is really important. Regular exercise has been a saviour. From a biological perspective, regular, moderate exercise can help reduce cortisol, which is a stress hormone, and boost serotonin, which makes you feel happy. There are also the instant effects of the release of endorphins during and post-workout. I like to listen to really loud rap music and do a pretty physical session to escape my thoughts and worries! But I actually feel the greatest difference over the following 24 hours. I always sleep much better if I've exercised that day, and I wake up in a better mood the following morning.

Moving forward, I've accepted that my life is always going to be extremely busy and unpredictable. I will always be worrying about something – I now worry about my creeping addiction to work and success and fear that the moment I relax everything will just disappear. I'm aware that onsets of anxiety can occur at any point, but the difference now is that I know that I don't have to lose power to it. I'm no longer scared. I'm taking charge of my health in a way I never have before and I surround myself with positive people. I don't usually have weekends off, so when I do have a day off filming, it is my 'me' day where I do all the things that make me feel good, whether it's buying myself flowers, having a sauna or eating pudding at a fancy restaurant. I say no to a lot more things – time is precious and I want to spend it wisely. You need time to make changes, start new relationships, explore new beginnings, look for a new job if your current one isn't making you happy. You can't let anxiety win the war: you have to acknowledge that it is there, but know that ultimately there are things you can do that can improve it. The tools opposite really help me cope with anxiety, and I hope they will help you too.

# my tools for coping with anxiety

1.  **Learn how to breathe properly.** Take a deep breath in through your nose, count to three, exhale through pursed lips.

2.  **Exercise regularly.** Choose happiness-inducing workouts. Try strength training, dancing or hiking. When I went through a break-up with Alik I started Zumba classes at my local gym, which I found exhilarating.

3.  **Keep busy.** Get out and do stuff. Find a new hobby to channel your energies.

4.  **Avoid relying on unhealthy crutches.** Don't use alcohol and other substances as a means to disengage the brain. Whilst alcohol might temporarily get rid of your anxiety, when it wears off the anxiety is likely to be much worse.

5.  **Find out what triggers your anxiety.** I now know my triggers, and no longer put myself in a position that I know is likely to cause anxiety.

6.  **Practise yoga.** Yoga is my go-to exercise to relax. Choose a class that combines physical poses with meditation and relaxation. Although I'm a very competitive sportswoman, what I love about yoga is that it is totally non-competitive – the idea is to practise at your own pace and develop your flexibility and strength.

7.  **Don't let your phone rule your life!** Lock it away for a few hours, stop mindlessly scrolling and have some real life conversations wherever possible, whether that be with a friend, the barista at your local café or a dog walker – you might just make someone's day!

8.  **Take time to physically relax and calm down.** Taking 15 minutes away from what you are doing when you have a surge of anxiety really helps.

9.  **Don't rely on caffeine when you're feeling down**. Caffeine kicks-starts the nervous system, but when under pressure all the nervous energy can cause an anxiety attack. I am very susceptible to the effects of caffeine, and sensitivity to it can increase at any point in your life, so don't think that it doesn't affect you just because you've been drinking five large lattes every day for the past 10 years. Switch to herbal tea instead.

10. **Get enough sleep.** Create a cosy, comfortable environment. Set aside enough time to sleep. Inconsistent or lack of sleep can contribute to overall stress, and this can turn into a vicious cycle because anxiety can make sleeping harder. (See page 37 for my sleep tips.)

11. **Don't skip meals.** If you feel nauseous then the last thing you will want to do is eat, so skipping meals might seem a good solution. But this will tamper with your blood sugar levels, which can make you feel worse.

12. **Focus on a goal.** This can be a good distraction – if you are going through an anxious phase then channel your energy into something positive, write a to-do list!

13. **Sharing is caring.** Talking to friends about your problems tends to make you feel better. I think you will be surprised by how many people suffer from similar thoughts at some stage in their life, so they should be able to relate to you. When you understand how normal it is, you'll feel less alone – we're in it together! Alternatively, writing a worry list or making a map of all of the things you're stressed by can be massively relieving.

14. **Walk!** It's easy, it's free and it's good for you! I try to walk as much as I can and have found it to be a great reliever to clear my head when I'm feeling panicked and nervous.

# rest well & get up early!

Forget the late nights, and prioritise sleep. After I threw in the party animal towel, I found the earlier I started going to bed, the earlier I would wake up and the better I would feel.

Sleep is imperative for proper cognitive function, optimal physical performance and the way we feel and look. Most sources suggest that between six and eight hours per night is the sweet spot for proper sleep but, as with diets and training methods, it depends on the individual. What works for you? If you run on more or less than eight hours, then great – but listen to your body. The aim is to wake each morning refreshed and revitalised, as if you've hit the reset button.

I always sleep with the curtains slightly open, because I like to wake up when it gets light. That way I can have the most productive day possible, with the additional benefit of soaking up the little bit of vitamin D that the UK has to offer. Because I like a 6am start, in the winter it means getting up before it gets light, but since I made changes to my lifestyle, I have definitely found this easier. When I was at my least healthy and happy, I would sometimes spend an entire day festering in bed. I now try to move as much as possible during the day and then have an early night; I'm usually in bed by 10pm at the latest. As you can probably imagine, early starts and early nights were almost unheard of for me before I turned my life around, but changing my sleep routine has been a big part of the transformation for me.

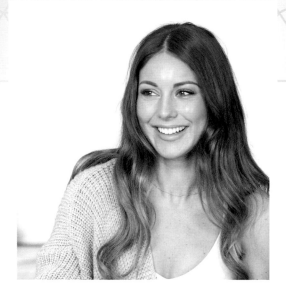

**Good diet and exercise goes a long way to improving your sleep, but here are some other tips that always help me get a peaceful night's rest:**

- **Drink herbal tea**, maybe chamomile or valerian, about 30–40 minutes before bed.

- **Ditch the electronics an hour before going to bed**, and don't take them into the bedroom with you. It's a distraction, and mobiles never sleep. They emit all sorts of radiation that are believed to stimulate our brains. Leave the phone outside the room, and let your brain switch off.

- **Read a few chapters of a good book**, or go through a very basic breathing pattern to calm your heart rate and in turn relax.

- **Change your bed sheets regularly**, and keep a clear, tidy bedroom. Clutter in the bedroom means clutter in the mind. De-clutter!

- **Wear something comfy.**

- **Have a warm, relaxing bath**, adding magnesium sulphate salts to the water.

- **Try to go to bed at the same time each night**, and try to wake up and get out of bed at the same time, every day. Difficult sometimes, I know, what with social schedules, illnesses etc. But if you can support what's called a circadian rhythm, whereby our body clock adjusts to knowing when it's time to power down and wake up again, so the engines get some proper rest, then the positive impact on getting proper sleep is fantastic.

- **Don't train too late in the day**, ideally no later than 6 or 7pm. If you exercise too late, it will kick-start the engines too much and this means it will take longer for you to fully relax.

- **An hour before bed, dim the lights in the room**. This will stimulate a natural secretion of melatonin – a hormone that is produced by the pineal gland, which regulates sleep and wakefulness. The more melatonin you are producing in the evening, the better your chance of a good sleep.

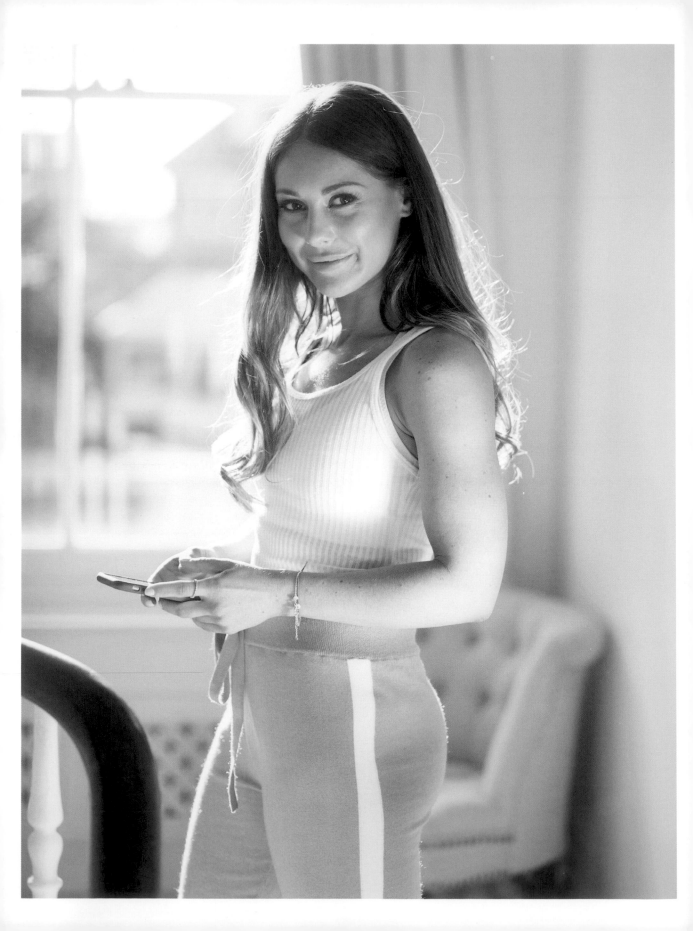

# how I feel now

I used to bulldoze my way through life with zero energy and no direction. Everything I do now is more slow and considered. This has been a change of attitude that has had a significant impact on all areas of my life. Life is about finding your own unique balance and path, and you are supposed to enjoy it along the way, appreciating all the small stuff that matters (that is often right in front of you). Seek out activities that lift you up, not drag you down.

For the first time ever I am in a stable place where I don't rely on anyone else to make me happy. And that puts me in a position where I can treat others properly – I am a firm believer that you have to be confident and content in yourself before you can treat someone else right. That is one of the main reasons why my relationship now is successful; I wasn't looking to get into it for the wrong reasons and I wasn't looking for a man to validate my sense of self-worth. My current boyfriend is a hero, but I don't rely on him. I owe Ryan for supporting me through a time where I dug deep to discover who I was and what I had to offer the world. He's given me some fantastic advice along the way and we bring out the best in one another.

It took a few repeat patterns before I learnt how to focus on the present and identify the things that I could change, that would improve my outlook and lead me to a better frame of mind. I have learnt that the only person who will ever be there 100 per cent for you is YOU. So put yourself first and look after yourself. I only surround myself with positive people who don't undermine me, but actually support me. Trust your instincts. I truly believe that you accept the love that you think you deserve. So set your standards high and good things will follow. Try not to regret and fixate on negative memories from the past. All mistakes teach us important lessons, and that's what I always have to remember too.

# staying motivated

I am guilty of procrastinating as much as the next person. I write to-do lists and then I won't follow through with things that I don't want to do, and they linger at the bottom of each new list I make. It happens time and time again, but now when it comes to things that I know help me to feel stronger and happier, I make the effort. It might be hard, but it is worth it, and that's a promise. Looking after yourself through moving more and eating well can seem quite self-centred, even selfish, but it's important. Remind yourself that it's a positive decision that can have profound effects on your health and outlook.

I try to remember that it's good for us to do something that we don't want to do each day to stay challenged and keep things different. I struggle with running, but this morning I forced myself to go on a run because the sun came out. I didn't set myself any strict targets but just ran (more like a jog) for 20 minutes. At around 10 minutes I thought I was going to pass out, then an inspirational image of a person I look up to popped into my head. I then thought about all the people who go through army training and ran a bit further. When I finished, I rewarded myself with a fresh juice and a lie down – if rewards work for kids then they work for me too!

It is better to do what you can with what you have than nothing at all. If the circumstances aren't right, then make them work. This is part of the reason that I've devised such simple workout plans (see pages 206–7) because I don't expect you to be able to leave the house after work when you have a family to feed and sort out or when you're dashing between other commitments. You'll be amazed by what is achievable using an inexpensive exercise mat at home. We can't help having days where we feel out of kilter, so on these days, or your lazy days, do the easy stuff. If you can muster the energy (reminding yourself that it is good for YOU) do something small – even if it's just going for a walk.

Find real food that tastes good to you. If you don't like something then don't just eat it for the sake of it. There are so many 'trendy' food types. First, the obsession was with avocado and then kale. Now it seems to be turmeric! Don't become fixated on the overload of new information or by eating the latest popular diet foods. There are loads of tasty, healthy foods, and you don't have to copy a certain food blogger or food trend.

Take an approach that fits YOUR lifestyle. If time or money present issues, or you're a crap cook, then be realistic. Your meals do not have to be gourmet, but that doesn't mean it's acceptable to head to the local fast-food joint. I've had times when my schedule has really interfered with my eating habits, leading to skipping meals and then eating HUGE amounts of food later on to make up for it. Because I am this way inclined I make sure I have healthy snacks around. I also cook extra portions at meal times so that I can take the rest in storage containers when I'm out all day. I used to think people who did this were a bit obsessive, but now I think it's genius.

I stay motivated by taking inspiration from other people. I have picked up a whole bunch of what I know from total strangers. People have shared with me what they do and what works for them, and there is no harm in giving things a go. And if you can find someone to exercise with it can be a bit more fun. Ryan, my brother Sam and I do ab exercises together and have a LOT of laughs. Sam always does it with his top off, which I find most offensive, but I have to agree that wearing minimal clothes at home can be effective because you can see where you are building strength. It's nice to be a part of something, and it can help you to stay motivated if you aren't always exercising alone. Whether you sign up for your local Park Run (a free, friendly 5k run at 9am every Saturday), or make friends at a nearby yoga class, I find that people who lean towards exercise tend to be friendly. You immediately have something in common. I've made a bunch of friends in my reformer Pilates class without even setting out to – I love speaking to my fellow students before the class starts and as we are packing up. We don't just talk about fitness – we share anecdotes about our families and weekend plans. All of this sociability helps no end with feeling energised.

 **It's important to do something that we don't want to do each day because that is a good way to stay challenged.**

One of the best things that Ryan has taught me since we've been together is not to be scared to stand up for what you believe in – the friends worth having will stick around, want what's best for you and respect the decisions you make through thick and thin. As I've navigated my way through my twenties, I have come to realise this more and more. Stick to your guns, and if the people around you are trying to lead you astray or don't think you're that fun anymore, drop them. I stopped trying to be cool a long time ago – I used to believe smoking was cool, that being invited to everything was cool or showing how much I could drink was cool. I can't believe how much I cared about 'cool'. Now I'm happy knowing I'm doing the right thing for me; I know my own mind, look after myself, and have confidence and belief in what I enjoy. This will make me feel better at the end of the day, and that's what motivates me.

We all have things to work on. Life is a journey of constant self-improvement. I know what I'm going to be working on moving into the future. I need to remember to keep taking it slow and make sure I enjoy the ride along the way. I often take things for granted, as my life moves at a quick pace, and I want to make sure it doesn't fly by without making time to cherish it.

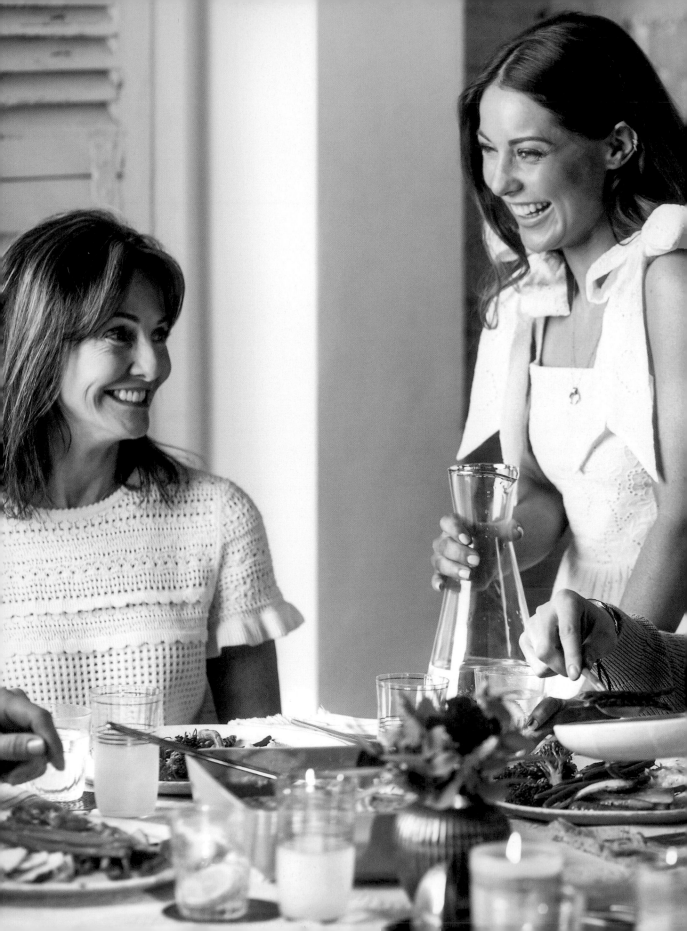

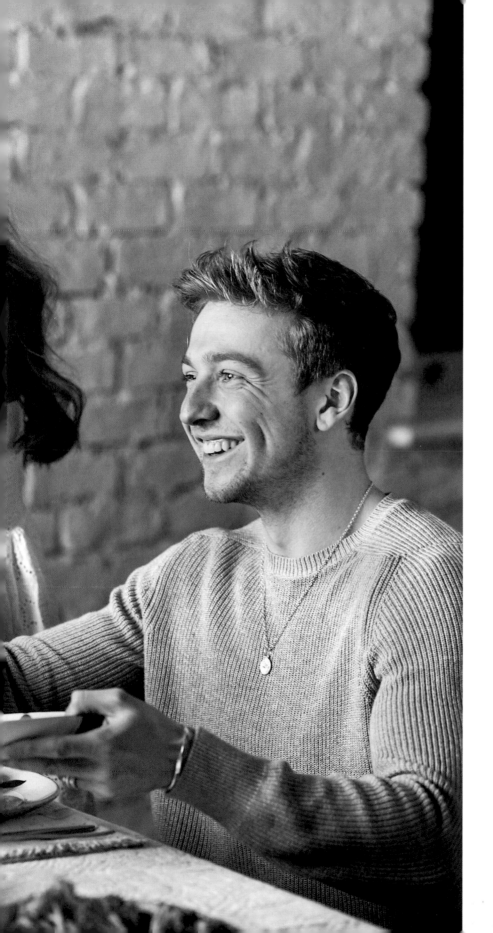

fall in love with food

PART 2

# how I eat now

Over the last couple of years, I've not just focussed on fitness; as I have taken steps to look after myself more, I've fallen back in love with food and cooking and all the joy it can bring to my day. I've tried countless faddy diets over the years, but *surprise surprise*, they never worked. And as anyone who knows me will confirm, I've always had a big appetite, so cutting down on calories left me pretty hangry and agitated. I now realise how damaging it is to restrict meals or to follow a fad diet made up of loads of rules. Denying yourself fuel is a recipe for unhappiness. I feel so guilty when I think back to my mum cooking me a delicious homemade spaghetti bolognese. I would only eat the sauce and leave the pasta on the side, thinking I was doing myself a favour. This habit of trying to eliminate carbs only left me starving later on in the day and inevitably reaching for sweets in my frantic search for an energy hit. I now don't cut out any entire food group, and allow everything in moderation. I hope my easy-going and relaxed ethos sounds refreshing.

I also used to be an absolute sucker for thinking things were healthy due to clever marketing. On reflection they weren't healthy at all, they were just fads, but I got sucked into the trap and used to go nuts for them. When I was studying at Edinburgh University I remember once filling two entire suitcases with 'healthy' smoothies and juices to take back on the train. I genuinely believed that I was going to turn into superwoman with all the nutrients I would get from these (sugar-heavy, I now realise) drinks, but the only benefit was the exercise that I got lugging them from A to B. I do occasionally have a juice or a smoothie (and on pages 166–69 I have included some of my favourites) because they come in handy for me when I am 'on the go' during a busy day of filming, but they shouldn't replace a proper meal.

It isn't rocket science to point out that the more you exercise, the more you need to eat. My primary goal is to feel better and achieve more in my day, and since I've started regularly exercising, I eat more than ever before and am in the strongest shape of my life. Cooking from scratch and using fresh ingredients means I have a solid understanding of how flavours work together and exactly what's going into my food. I'm super excited to share my favourite recipes and I hope this shows that cooking tasty food doesn't need to be hard – plenty of the recipes I've included can also be prepared in advance, frozen and taken to work with you to be eaten cold the next day. Now that I have a bank of quick core recipes, I'm constantly expanding on them by adding new ingredients and different toppings, testing them out on Sam and Ryan. One of my best discoveries is my banana and chocolate pancakes (see pages 66–67). I never imagined that pancakes would one day be good for you but this sort of thing puts a massive smile on my face.

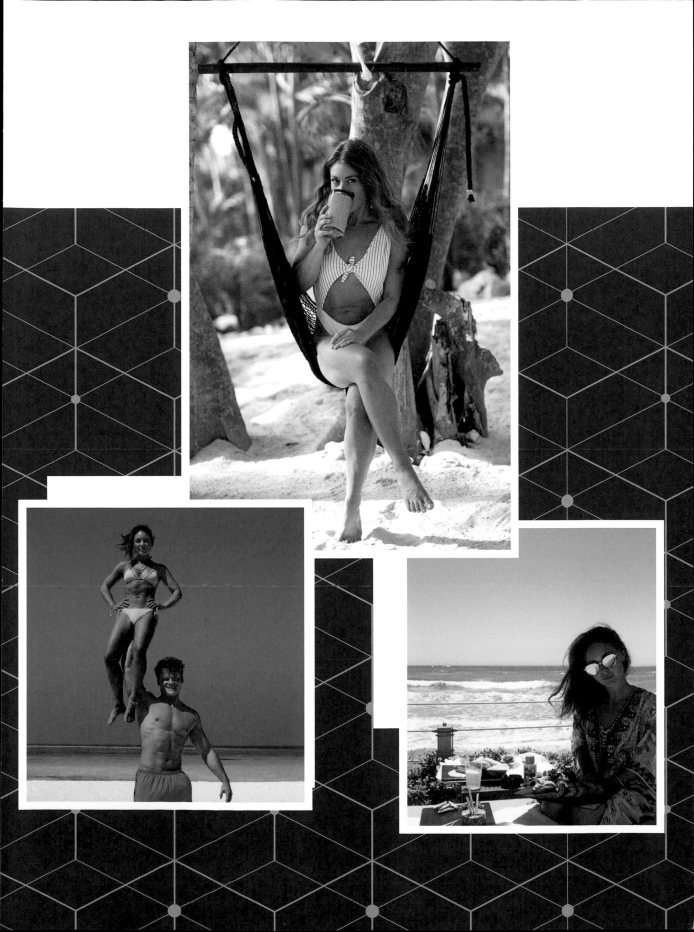

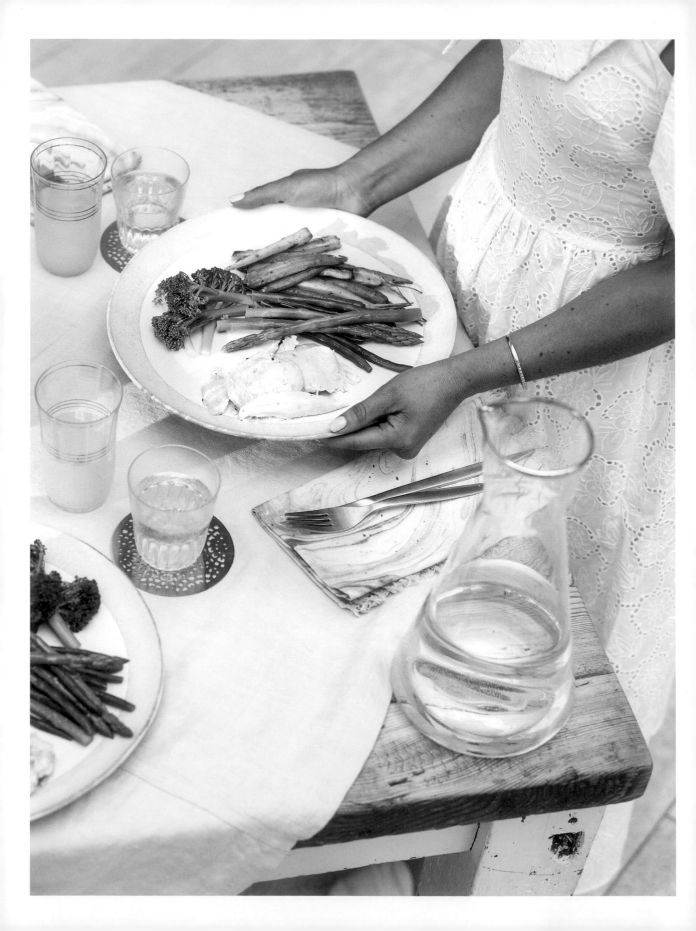

I never know when or where I'm going to end up eating, but it's a priority for me to try to cook at home whenever I can, slowing down to enjoy that time. Most of you reading this book will probably follow a more structured daily routine than I do, so you might find it a bit easier to plan your meals. I want you to look forward to mealtimes and get creative with them. However, equally important are the times when you are out and about or busy and don't know how you are going to be able to fit it all in. It's good to try to adapt to these situations and not throw all of your dedication out of the window. The occasional slip-up isn't a problem of course, but a little dedication to eating well at least 80 per cent of the time is required. If you want change you do have to make time for it – but the benefits can be amazing. I certainly prioritise mealtimes and workouts over other things now because I have found that the knock-on effect is that I am happier and more energised that way.

In general, my approach is to eat food with nutritional benefit. I combatted my cravings for unhealthy snacks by being open-minded about options that were better for me, and now I truly prefer the taste of lower-sugar foods. If I'm craving something crunchy and tasty, instead of crisps I'll make a batch of my favourite dips – see pages 176–177 – and snack on that or home-made vegetable crisps, or dried sugar snap peas or chickpea crisps, which are far less addictive. Once you combat the cravings, substituting healthier alternatives becomes easier. You'll find ideas for more of my favourite healthy snacks on page 54.

Since I was little I've always loved cooking for myself, and more recently I have started cooking regularly for my friends, family and boyfriend. I was lucky enough to do a Leith's cookery course while I was at school, but now I've developed more of an experimental style of cooking which is more practical and less time-consuming. The kitchen is one of the few areas where I seem to liberate my over-controlling and perfectionist personality, so I embrace it with open arms!

On the following pages, there are plenty of super-quick meals that you can cook up post-workout or, if you are working out at lunchtime, that you can prepare the night before and take into work in storage containers. To make things easy, some of the recipes in this section have little symbols that tell you if a dish is good for post-workout, is one I regularly serve up when I'm entertaining guests or is a meal I pack up to take with me when I'm out all day.

# putting together a plate of food

I'm not claiming to be a food scientist or nutritionist, but I do try to stay informed. I also make a point of listening to my body and responding to what it needs. For example, I've learnt that I don't digest red meat as well as other meats, so I aim not to eat it more than a couple of times a week. But it's important to work out what best suits you; we are all so different and lead such different lives. I've also found that for MY metabolism I shouldn't go longer than 5 hours without having something to eat because that way I'm less likely to reach for the sweets when my blood sugar has dropped.

I was brought up to finish all the food on my plate, and although it's a good idea to gauge in advance how much you will eat to avoid waste, you shouldn't feel you have to finish everything. My eyes used to be far too big for my stomach and I would always load more food onto my plate than I needed. Remember that you can always go back for second helpings, but try to leave it 20 minutes and the chances are you will feel satisfied after all.

I also grew up surrounded by boys in my family. My appetite was always pretty big and I would eat three-course dinners on the regular with my dad and brother. Then, later on, when spending time with whichever boyfriend I was with, I would notice that I picked up their habits – I am a sucker for eating similar amounts to whoever I'm at lunch or dinner with. My current partner Ryan eats six large meals a day in order to keep his body looking the way it does. Of course, the more you exercise the more you need to refuel because you burn through it a lot quicker. However, if I ate the same amount of calories as Ryan does then I would balloon. When we first started dating, I would eat more because it was social spending mealtimes together. Now I've learnt I have to be selfish and so I make sure I eat to suit my needs and on my timescale – although we do always stick to our obligatory Sunday roast, where people find it shocking that Ryan and I eat the same amount of food!

In recent years, carbohydrates have got a bad reputation, but I would never recommend avoiding them altogether: not only are they crucial to your diet, but it's unrealistic to think you will manage to cut them out completely. I just try to avoid refined and processed carbs where beneficial fibre has been stripped away, such as white bread and white rice. In exchange, I eat complex carbs that absorb slowly into your system. These take the form of vegetables, whole fruits, legumes, whole grains and seeds. In a restaurant I try not to fill up on bread before the meal. In fact, I usually avoid it being put on the table, unless it's a tasty olive focaccia or some fresh sourdough!

I like to get as much colour onto my plate as possible at every meal, not least because a range of colour indicates a healthy balance of nutrients. Typically, when plating up a meal I visualise the plate in quarters, aiming for a good balance of carbohydrates, fats and protein. I aim to fill half the plate with colourful vegetables or salad (even adding some fruit), and then a quarter with a complex (wholegrain) carbohydrate, and the remaining quarter with a lean protein. It tends to work with most of the meals I like to eat, and even when I've made something like a big pie, I will make sure when it comes to serving that the veg portion makes up half the plate. I don't think you can go wrong with this rule! I have to say I'm even starting to enjoy vegetables more in the morning, one of my favourites being leftover vegetable omelette (see pages 74–75).

 **My post-training meal is the one I look forward to the most! If I've done a high-intensity workout that included some cardio then I will ramp up my carbohydrate serving in this meal.**

Typically I have a small(ish) breakfast if I'm doing a morning workout because I don't like to exercise on a full stomach. Then I make sure to have a good-sized lunch and dinner. Honestly, my post-training meal is the one I look forward to the most. If I've done a high-intensity workout that included some cardio then I will ramp up my carbohydrate serving in this meal. If you want to build muscle then aim to eat more protein and carbohydrate post-workout than you would usually, to help rebuild the muscle effectively. In the past when I've limited my carb intake post-workout, thinking it might benefit my body, I've noticed it has a negative effect on my energy levels.

Protein is important for building muscle – and also keeping our bones and skin healthy – but as with any element of your diet, you need to be selective. I've always been a big meateater, but I choose leaner types and cuts of meat, such as poultry, which is also lower in fat than darker meats such as beef, lamb or pork (although this is dependent on the cut, and removing the skin when cooking chicken will cut down on saturated fat). I also aim to get my protein from other non-meat sources (and cutting back on red meat also happens to be a sound environmental move), including beans, lentils and pulses, quinoa, eggs, milk, cheese, yoghurt, seafood, soya, tempeh, buckwheat, mycoprotein and nuts – and of course there is loads of variation in protein levels within these. The good news is that most protein-rich foods are bought in their natural state so you can easily eliminate eating processed foods if you want to adopt a protein-rich diet.

I aim to eat fish a few times a week so that I can benefit from the lean source of protein and from the omega-3 fatty acids, which are great for my hair, skin and nails. White fish is almost always low in fat, but it's the fatty fish, such as salmon, which contains the omega-3 beneficial fats. Why would I take expensive supplements when I know that a good diet can be sufficient?

Eggs in any form make a great, quick meal, so I eat a lot of them and always have some at home. Although we've been led to believe that eggs are heavy in cholesterol, I have read that eating saturated and trans fats, combined with too many refined carbs and sugars, is far more likely to raise your cholesterol levels than eating foods that have a high cholesterol content in themselves.

Don't be scared of fats. Although frying and roasting in lots of butter and oil or eating loads of creamy or cheesy sauces isn't going to be doing you any favours, polyunsatured fats, found in seeds, vegetable oils (especially the cold-pressed ones) and fatty fish (such as trout and salmon) are good for your heart. Monounsaturated fats, found in olive oil, avocados and most nuts, are also good for you in moderation – they are quite high in calories and although I don't count calories, I am mindful of this when it comes to even healthy fats, as they can quickly add up. You'll see in my recipes that I tend to use butter or olive oil for cooking and save my cold-pressed, extra-virgin oils for drizzles and dressings.

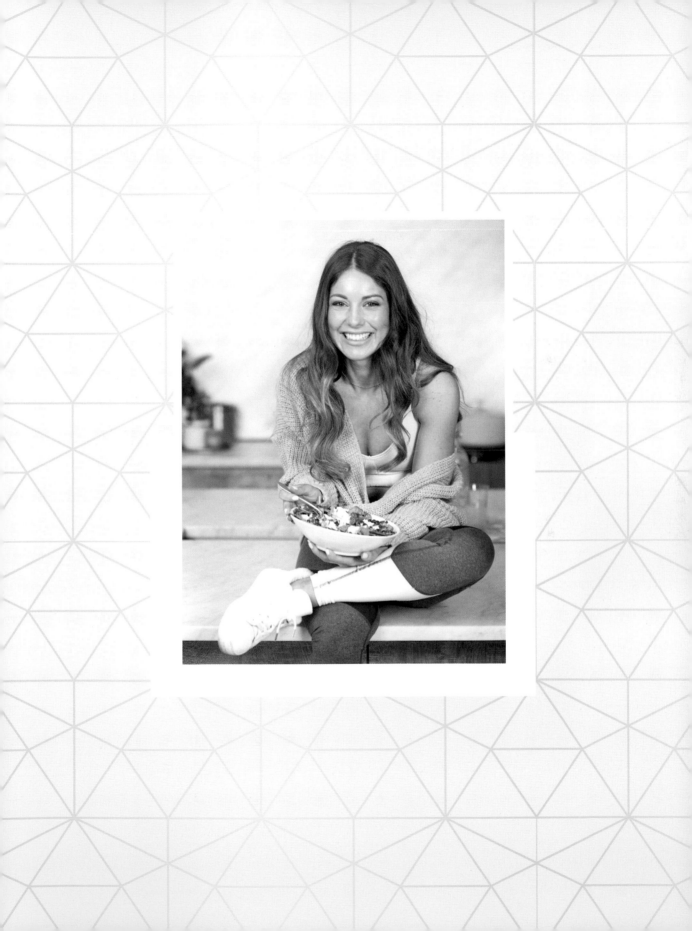

# drink enough water

Drinking enough water is clearly vital. Our bodies rely on fluid to operate properly, and being dehydrated can lead to a whole host of problems. I like to drink at least 2 litres a day, or roughly 8 glasses. Of course, it depends on your body size and weight and how much you move around (as well as the weather!), so this is just a guideline. I used to be really useless at keeping hydrated, but now I make it a priority and always carry a refillable water bottle around with me. A good way to make sure you fulfil your daily standard is by drinking enough in the morning before you leave the house and at night before bed – it can be easy to forget during the day, especially if you're busy. Something I've learnt is that you don't have to wait until you feel thirsty to drink water. Feeling thirsty is a sign that you are already dehydrated, so you should drink it whenever you can find a chance or if you haven't had a glass of water for at least an hour.

Since making an active decision to drink at least 8 glasses of water a day, I have noticed that I have more energy as well as a really healthy and active digestive system. I have also had compliments on my skin. If you don't drink enough water you are likely to feel tired, and you might feel hungry because your body thinks it needs food for energy – sometimes your body can mistake thirst for hunger, and rather than a snack, all you actually need is a glass of water to hit the spot. So resist that 4pm sugar hit and reach for a glass of water instead, wait for 20 minutes to see how you feel.

# a note on alcohol

As I've already discussed my relationship with alcohol, I'm sure it comes as no surprise that I rarely drink it now, bar the occasional glass of red wine with a roast lunch on a Sunday or over a meal with friends, or a gin and tonic when out with friends. I find white and rosé wine too acidic (maybe I drank too much of it in my teenage years...) and I definitely avoid mixing my drinks. Just as with my food choices, I avoid anything that is loaded with sugar or secret ingredients, so fancy cocktails are a straight-up no... with the exception of an espresso martini because I adore the taste of coffee!

I take a lot of inspiration from Ryan, who also barely drinks alcohol, and you only have to look at him to see the shape that he is in. I have found that if I do have drinks the night before I exercise, then I'm not able to perform at my maximum capacity when training the next day. Cutting right down was something I needed to do in my life generally, and now I can really see the benefit this has on my workouts and mental wellbeing too.

In terms of training, alcohol has damaging effects on all the factors that we need to gain muscle, such as hydration and recovery, and negatively affects the absorption of most nutrients, including protein. Protein absorption is needed for anabolism (the building process) to take place, and if you aren't absorbing protein then your muscle tissue can't repair itself as quickly. Muscle building takes place by breaking down muscle fibres and then subsequently rebuilding the damaged tissue, so it is pretty essential that you encourage anabolism as much as possible. In short, what this means is that consuming alcohol regularly is likely to reduce lean muscle mass.

As we know, a lot of our performance during workouts comes from being in the right headspace – you need a positive mind to reap positive rewards. When I drink alcohol, I know it takes at least 24 hours for the alcohol to fully clear my system and for my brain function to return to normal. As I get older I truly feel the effects last longer, and getting my ass into gear and walking to the gym is the last thing on my mind when all I want to do is just survive the day with minimal interaction. I guarantee your workout will feel better when you're not suffering a one- or two-day hangover.

# snacking

I don't think it's a problem to snack during the day. As I've said before, I like to eat when I'm hungry, and I don't like being hungry, so as long as you're not just eating for the sake of it, then go ahead. I think the most important thing is to have healthy snack options to hand. When you get hunger cravings, the last thing you want to do is spend time preparing things or scraping around for healthy ideas. It might sound trivial, but as a busy person I'm faced with this battle every day. When I get home starving I go straight to the fridge and open up the top flap on the door to see if there is any dark chocolate. Then I go for one of the drawers, have a quick scout around the shelves, then I'll check the store cupboard and the pull-out drawers. If I can't find anything healthy, I freak out and will eat anything I can get my hands on out of desperation. So line up some healthy choices and keep them stocked up. Plus, if you're training a lot then you need to make sure you are keeping fuelled throughout the day.

## some of my favourite snacks

- **Mixed unsalted nuts, especially almonds and pistachios**
- **Apple quarters with peanut butter**
- **Satsumas**
- **Kale chips** – these are so easy to make; coat the kale in oil, sprinkle with salt, then roast on a tray in the oven at 140°C/120°C fan/gas 1 for 10–15 minutes.
- **Small amounts of dark chocolate**
- **Cucumber with hummus**
- **Corncakes with avocado**
- **A hard-boiled egg**
- **Edamame beans**
- **Olives**
- **Sun-dried tomatoes**
- **Popcorn**
- **Rye bread with crumbled feta**
- **Cooked prawns**
- **Frozen grapes** (they taste like ice lollies!)

# how to balance a social life with eating well

I make sure I throw the BEST dinner parties so I don't miss out on having a social life. I invite my friends who I owe favours to and cook a three-course meal, with big sharing dishes – I've included some of my entertaining recipes in this book so you can try them too. For Christmas last year my dad gave me money to take out a few of my friends for a meal and I thought this was the nicest idea ever. I've learnt to value experiences over owning things, and have found the satisfaction I used to get from acquiring new things doesn't compete with that of creating memories. I have taken material goods for granted at times, so have spent time over the past year clearing out the stuff that I used to collect by giving it to charity. Nothing beats a dinner party with good food and good friends. That is irreplaceable.

I have such fond memories of my dad cooking the most MEGA roasts on the weekend. It was a big deal within our family because it was one of the only times we would all get together, especially given that I was away from home from the age of 11 and Sam from 8. Dad would pile our plates high with meat, veggies and the biggest Yorkshire puddings I've ever seen. The entire kitchen would be in action with loads of saucepans bubbling away on the hob. The word spread around school and I used to have requests from friends to come over for Sunday lunch to assess the mountainous portions. Growing up eating this traditional British fodder is probably what led to my obsession with cooking my own roast dinners, which has turned into a bit of a contest! I give a rating to each one I prepare, comparing overall size, potato fluffiness, richness of gravy, different trimmings... the list goes on. I definitely take inspiration from my dad, but I definitely cook with less butter than he does.

I am aware that a roast isn't the most healthy option, but this furthers my point that balance is important. Like most things in life, eating is all about compromise. There are ways in which you can make it a bit healthier, for example eating a lean cut of meat, or by not adding fat to the gravy. Perhaps the most important factor is remembering the plating up rule, and making sure a large portion of your meal is made up of delicious roast vegetables.

When it comes to eating out, I make a decision between a starter or a pudding. I used to overeat in restaurants and it would make me lethargic and almost uncomfortable in my clothes. I try to remember this when I'm ordering food, choosing something that's better for me, rather than just whatever everyone else is having.

# keeping a food diary

Although I am really against becoming obsessive about any aspect of life, keeping a food diary can be a good idea if only as a temporary experiment, because you will learn a lot about what you consume. Many of the things that we eat or drink we disregard or don't even notice we are consuming. The more mindful you are about what is going into your body, the more quickly you will notice the benefits. If you're going to invest time into doing this then you might as well note down the exercises you are doing too, so you can have a better understanding of your food and fitness balance. Then you can work out whether one has an impact on the other. There are loads of apps to help with recording this sort of thing.

The main benefits of keeping a food diary are learning what food groups you are lacking. You will learn quickly whether there are foods that you are avoiding and then you can figure out ways to incorporate them so that you have a balanced diet. It is not a calorie-counting venture. What you are aiming for is to eat three balanced meals. Make sure to really listen to your body. You are likely to learn what foods you eat and crave at different times of the day. If you find yourself constantly craving something to eat at 3pm, maybe think about changing what you eat at lunchtime so you stay fuller for longer. If you are following my mantra of only eating when you're hungry, you will learn a lot. You may find you're not that hungry during the day and light meals work best for you, and that you like to have a bigger meal in the evening. Or maybe you prefer a larger breakfast but then lighter meals for the rest of the day. It's not necessarily about when you are eating but about the food that you choose to eat. For me, when I'm having a lazy evening I can eat more heavy foods because then I'm just going to be unwinding, relaxing and sleeping – I tend to do my exercise in the morning. If you can only work out later on in the day, avoid having a super-heavy lunch because you will feel a lot less motivated when you're really full.

If you feel that writing it down doesn't fit into your hectic schedule then you can easily take a picture as a reminder. You might be surprised at how often you find you are getting your phone out of your pocket. I've recently had Invisalign braces and the number of times that I had to take them out to eat proved to me how frequently I was snacking, and occasionally made me question whether I was actually hungry or not. I do the same for my progress at the gym: if I'm using any of the cardio machines I will take a photo to track my progress with distances, inclines and times, as a positive reminder. I also love taking photos of all my food creations and particularly pretty meals to remind me how much I love cooking when I'm having a difficult day and am not feeling very inspired.

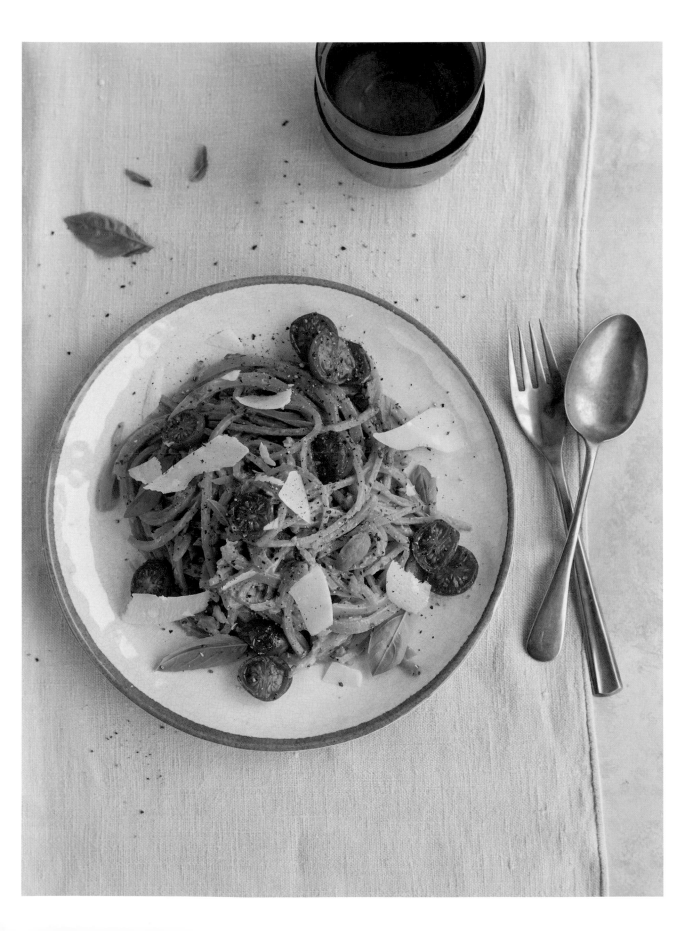

# food and fitness: my week at a glance

I love seeing what foodie concoctions others are whipping up in their kitchens along with the workouts people are trying, so here's my typical week in food and fitness in case anyone shares my curiosity. I don't cook anything too complicated, but focus on simple meals from scratch using fresh ingredients, especially when time is short. My schedule changes from week to week, but I try to stick to three meals a day with one or two snacks.

## monday

**7am**
Home workout (see pages 206–207)

**8am**
Breakfast Stir-Fry (see page 86)

**11am**
A hard-boiled egg

**1pm**
Chicken Caesar Salad (see page 96)

**7pm**
Tofu with steamed broccoli and sweet potato mash
(*I microwave my sweet potato to speed up cooking*)

## tuesday

**8am**
My Protein Porridge (see page 73)

**11am**
Dark chocolate-covered rice cakes

**1.30pm**
Lunch meeting at a delicious Asian-fusion restaurant. I ate several tasting dishes, including duck salad, crunchy sushi and miso aubergine

**7.30pm**
Easy Flatbread Pizza (see page 152)

## wednesday

**7am**
Matcha and Chia Seed Overnight Pudding (see page 76)

**11am**
Home workout (see pages 206–207)

**12.30pm**
Salmon fillet with wilted greens

**3pm**
Blueberry Burst Slices (see page 171)

**7pm**
Baked Sweet Potatoes with Bean Chilli, Guacamole & Greek Yoghurt (see page 150)

## thursday

**7.30am**
Banana and Chocolate 'Everything Free' Pancakes (see page 66)

**1pm**
Mozzarella Salad with Broad Beans, Peas, Mint and a Lemony Dressing, taken in lunchbox (see page 92)

**3pm**
Bag of salted popcorn and a Green Smoothie (see page 92)

**7.30pm**
Spicy Prawn Laksa (see page 137)

## YES, I am trying to eat well. NO, I am not on a diet.

I aim to eat a balanced diet that gives me energy and helps me feel my best; but you will notice that I don't 'restrict' myself which is why this is NOT an intimidating food diary. Check out my recipes and let me know how you get on!

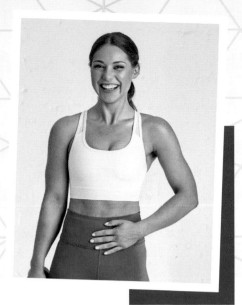

## friday

**8am**
Workout session in the gym – you can easily do my home workout plans on the gym mat too! (See pages 206–207)

**9.30am**
Two poached eggs on fresh sourdough

**2.30pm**
My Pack-Up-and-Go Chicken Pho (see page 120)

**4pm**
Crudités and Dips (see page 177)

**7pm**
Roasted Carrot Farro Salad with Kale, Goat's Cheese & Walnuts (see page 161) and a bowl of Yoghurt with Protein Powder for pudding (see page 178)

## saturday

**9am**
Reformer Pilates class

**10.30pm**
Strawberry Porridge with Flaked Almonds & Pumpkin seeds (see page 69) and a protein shake

**1pm**
Butternut Squash Soup (see page 100)

**3pm**
Slice of Courgette Loaf (see page 172)

**8pm**
I cooked a dinner party for six friends. For the starter I served my Courgette, Walnut & Ricotta Quiche with a Quinoa Crust (see page 112), then for the main event I cooked Easy Spicy Chicken Thighs & Colourful Veg Tray Bake (see page 144)

## sunday

**9.30am**
I cooked Scrambled Eggs with Roasted Herby Tomatoes, Green Leaves & Home-made Beans (see page 83) for me, my boyfriend and my brother, and I served it with slices of the Courgette Loaf (see page 172) that I baked on Saturday

**2.30pm**
Blueberry Burst Slice (see page 171)

**5pm**
This is more like 'linner'. On Sundays my family are dedicated to our roast ritual. This Sunday, I made my One-tray Roast Chicken with Lower-fat Dauphinoise Potatoes (see pages 124–127) and I look forward to feasting on the leftovers for a cheerful Monday lunch

# don't beat yourself up!

I don't like to restrict anything. I never say never, because then you are setting yourself up for failure. My approach to food doesn't mean that I never eat chocolate, for example. If I was at a friend's house or at a birthday party I would rarely say no to a slice of cake because I don't want to make a point of being on some fancy diet or draw attention to it. That defeats the point of it, and how bored are people going to get of constantly hearing about your food requirements and how well your diet is going? VERY.

I never struggle with saying no to things or feeling guilty or hungry anymore, because I have learnt to make more informed choices and have steered myself clear of the dangerous path of obsessive eating. I have healthy weeks followed by a few slip-ups or treats. It's about balance. As long as I don't set myself unrealistic challenges then I don't feel I'm struggling to stick to anything. I prefer making small changes that I can stick to, for example my recent push for more vegetables at breakfast time. As I introduce more of these mini changes, I notice the overall picture improving. I know that I am at the top of my game with regards to my strength, and although I do fluctuate month to month I know that I will never fall into the unhealthy patterns I was in before. I've come way too far. I used to think that you had to be strict to see results, but the proof is in the pudding: you can still your dream body while eating your 'guilty' pleasures.

One of the biggest lessons I've learnt on my journey is to just be me. Most of us make comparisons to other people without even realising we are doing it and this can contribute to insecurities and unhappiness especially when it comes to food. I used to think it was positive to look at other people for inspiration on what to look like, to motivate and encourage me, but ultimately the moment I started focusing on myself and stopped worrying about what other people were up to, I became quite liberated. I accept that there are things that I can change, and there are things that I cannot change, so I'm going to do the best with what I've got. We all have strengths and weaknesses in different areas, and this applies to food too. Different things will suit different bodies, including different eating habits and patterns, and we all struggle in different ways with different parts of our body, which is why it's so important to pay attention. Listen to your body, learn what it needs and treat it with the respect it deserves.

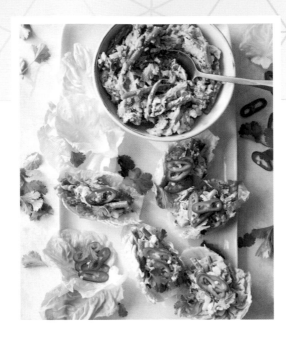

## my **top 10** mantras for healthy eating

- Enjoy your food! Experiment in the kitchen and cook meals from scratch.

- Make sure you have healthy food options in your kitchen. Don't fill your cupboards with junk.

- Eat regularly. Don't let yourself get too hungry or, worse still, hangry!

- Sit down at a table to eat. And not in front of the television. Whenever I eat standing up or am distracted/multi tasking I don't get the satisfaction of sitting down with the sole purpose of enjoying a meal. My brain doesn't seem to register that I've eaten and I tend to graze all afternoon or evening as a result.

- Don't worry about slipping up. The occasional treat isn't going to derail all your good work so don't beat yourself up about the odd biscuit or indulgent meal out. Enjoy it!

- Drink plenty of water. Cut out fizzy drinks and alcohol.

- Eat when you are hungry and stop when you are full. This sounds simple but it's easy to overeat.

- Sleep more. OK, this is more of a lifestyle tip but if you have enough sleep you will be more in tune with your body.

- Stop ordering takeaways. It is such a waste of money.

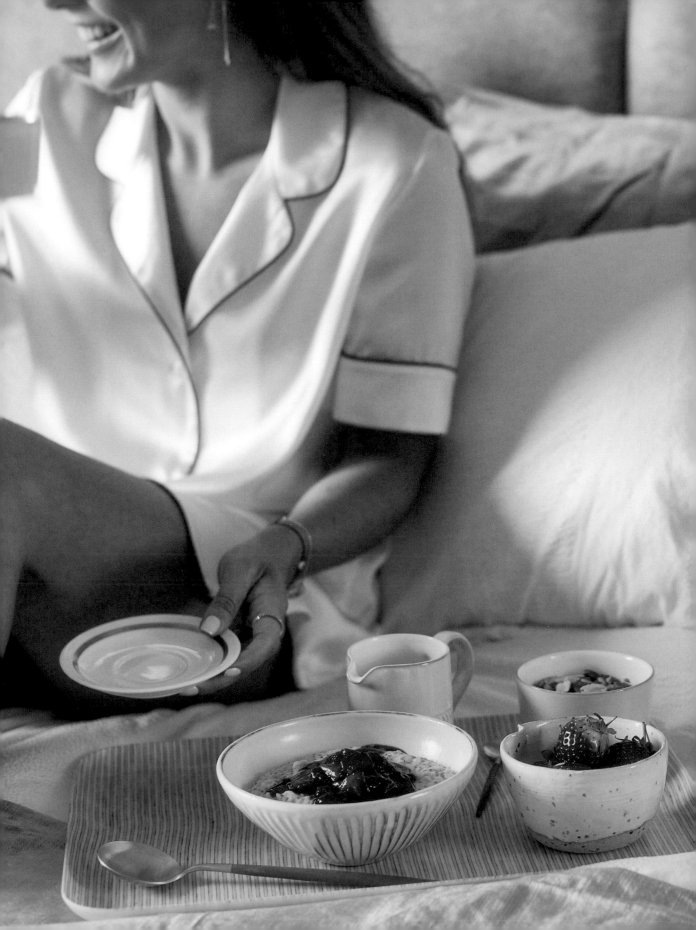

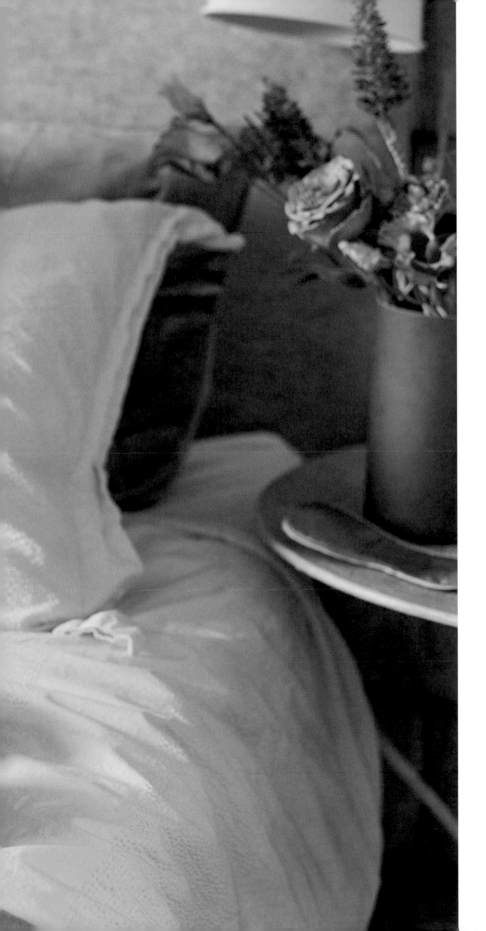

breakfast
& brunch

# kale & sweet potato hash with poached eggs & avocado

I LOVE the combination of a runny egg yolk with crunchy potato first thing in the morning. I like to prepare batches of potato hash and put them in the freezer ready to defrost them overnight in the fridge to speed up my breakfast prep.

## serves 2

2 sweet potatoes, peeled and grated (about 250g)

2 tsp olive oil

1 red onion, finely chopped

2 spring onions, finely sliced

1 garlic clove, finely chopped

1 red chilli, finely chopped (*optional*)

40g kale, leaves torn and tough stalks removed

½ tsp smoked paprika

3 medium eggs

a splash of white wine vinegar (*optional*)

½ avocado, sliced

1 tbsp finely chopped chives

salt and black pepper

Preheat the oven to 200°C/180°C fan/gas 6 and line a baking tray with non-stick baking paper.

Squeeze the grated sweet potato to remove as much liquid as possible and place in a mixing bowl. This is important as otherwise you will end up with soggy hash! Heat 1 teaspoon of the olive oil in a frying pan over a medium heat and sauté the red onion, spring onions, garlic and chilli, if using, for 3 minutes. Add the torn kale leaves and continue to cook for another 2–3 minutes until the kale has wilted.

Remove from the heat and add to the bowl with the sweet potato. Add the smoked paprika and season to taste. Crack one of the eggs into a small bowl, beat it and then stir into the mixture until everything is well combined.

Divide the mixture into 4 and shape into rounds using your hands. Place on the lined baking tray, drizzle with the remaining olive oil and bake for 18–20 minutes, until cooked through and golden brown.

Before the potato hash is ready, bring a large saucepan of water up to simmering point. Add a splash of white wine vinegar if you have it. Crack the remaining 2 eggs into separate cups or ramekins. Swirl the water and then carefully tip one egg, followed by the other, into the hot water to the side of the pan. Reduce the heat to a gentle simmer and poach for 3 minutes for soft eggs, then remove with a slotted spoon and drain on kitchen paper.

Stack two sweet potato cakes on each serving plate, top with the avocado slices and a poached egg. Sprinkle over the chopped chives and serve immediately.

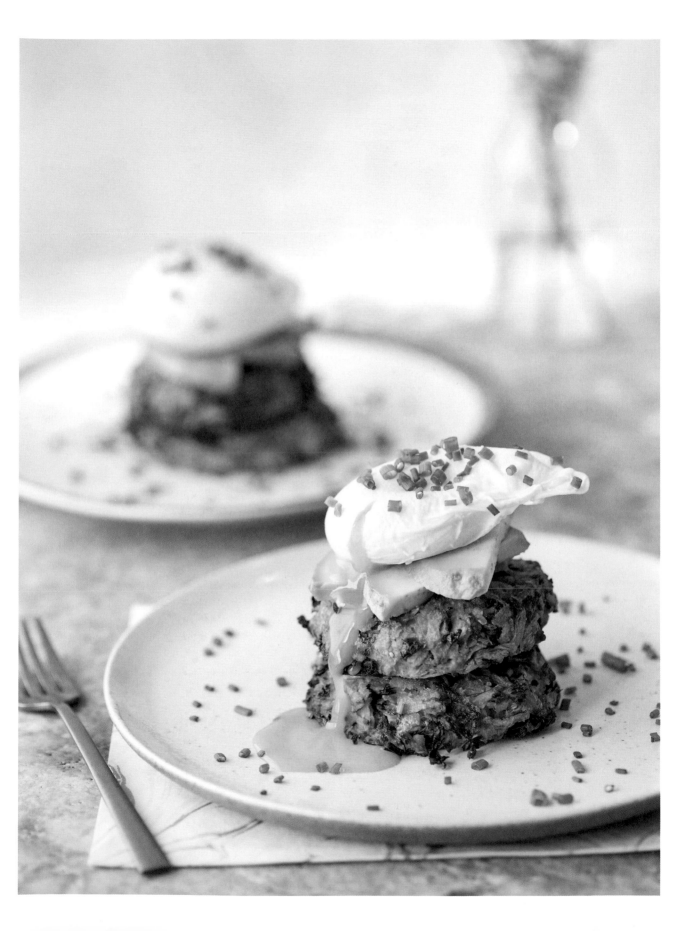

# banana & chocolate 'everything-free' pancakes

When I first discovered a recipe for pancakes that consisted of just banana, eggs and cocoa powder I assumed it would taste revolting. It didn't and I was flabbergasted by how light and fluffy they came out. Now I make these all the time, adding whatever toppings suit my mood.

## serves 4
### (makes 8 pancakes)

2 large, ripe bananas

2 tbsp unsweetened cocoa powder (or a vegan chocolate protein powder)

2 large eggs

1 tbsp light olive oil

100g coconut yoghurt (or fat-free Greek yoghurt if you eat dairy)

80g frozen berries

20g toasted flaked almonds

a handful of mint leaves, to garnish

Roughly chop the bananas into a mixing bowl and use a fork to mash them into a purée. Using electric beaters, beat in the cocoa powder or protein powder. Add an egg and beat into the mix. Repeat for the second egg then continue to whisk everything together for 2–3 minutes until the mixture increases in volume and becomes pale and airy.

Heat the oil in a frying pan over a medium heat. Drop in spoonfuls of the pancake batter – this will make 8 small pancakes and you will probably need to cook them in batches. Cook for 4–5 minutes until bubbles start to appear on the surface, the pancakes are cooked underneath and they hold their shape well, then carefully turn them over (they are more delicate than regular flour-based pancakes) and cook for 1 minute on the other side. Remove from the pan and stack on your serving plates.

Top each pancake stack with Greek yoghurt, frozen berries and flaked almonds. Add a few mint leaves and serve immediately.

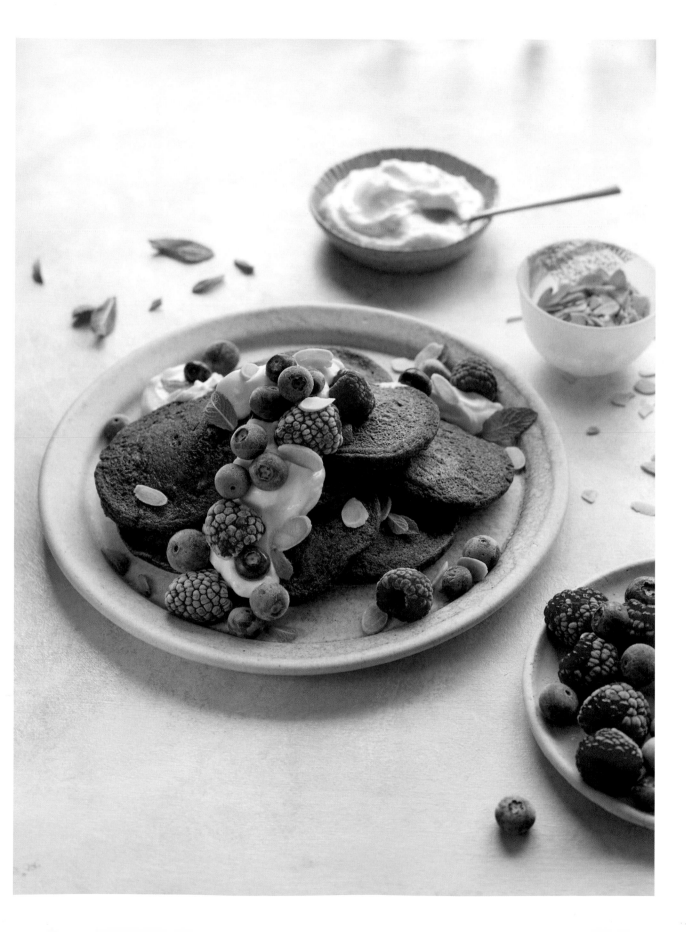

# porridge three ways

I didn't buy into porridge until fairly recently because I always favoured a fry up. Now I get the same amount of satisfaction from these comforting bowls of goodness. What I love about porridge is you can jazz it up with so many diverse flavours. My protein porridge is great if you prefer to eat something savoury in the morning. *(See next page for photograph.)*

### The base grain:

You can pretty much use any of the following as the base for your porridge. I like keeping all of these in my cupboard to mix it up from time to time, or even combine them together.

- Rolled oats (oatmeal)
- Barley flakes
- Buckwheat flakes
- Spelt flakes
- Quinoa
- Chia seeds
- Milled flaxseed

### The liquid:

Similarly, you can choose which liquid you would like to make it with. This is down to personal preference. Each will offer a different flavour, texture, nutritional benefit and calorie count.

- Water
- Cow's milk
- Almond milk
- Coconut milk

### The toppings:

The great thing about porridge is you can experiment with different flavour combinations to make it more exciting. These are some of my favourites:

- Blackberry and apple with honey

- Banana, blueberry, flaked almonds & cinnamon

- Raspberry, coconut & poppy seeds or flaxseeds

- Cocoa, peanut butter, pecans & bananas

- Dark chocolate & dates

- Yoghurt, maple syrup & pomegranate seeds

serves 1

## basic porridge

50g base grain
250ml liquid

Bear in mind that different grains absorb different amounts of liquid, so use these measures as a starting point only, adding more or less liquid as needed and according to your preference.

Add the base grain and liquid to a saucepan. Cook over a medium-low heat for around 4–5 minutes, stirring frequently once it's started steaming so that it doesn't stick to the bottom of the pan.

If you want your porridge runnier, add a little more liquid until you get the consistency that you like.

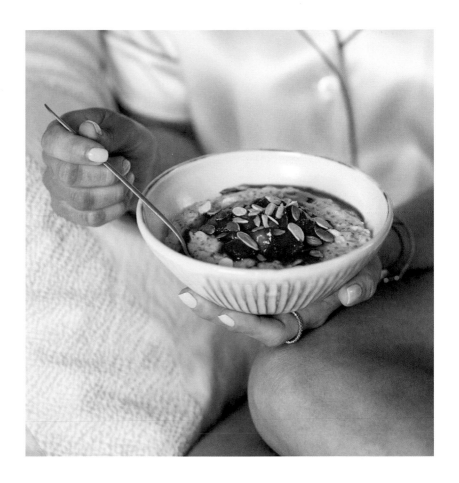

## strawberry porridge with flaked almonds & pumpkin seeds

### serves 2
75g rolled oats
25g barley flakes
1 tbsp chia seeds
200ml almond milk
300ml water

### for the topping
200g strawberries
1 tbsp maple syrup
15g toasted flaked almonds
1 tbsp pumpkin seeds

Add the oats, barley flakes and chia seeds to a small saucepan along with the almond milk and water. Place on a medium–low heat. While this is starting to cook, roughly chop the strawberries. Put them in another small saucepan with the maple syrup. Place over a high heat and cook for about 3 minutes to make a super-quick compote. Remove from the heat to cool slightly.

Stir the porridge regularly once it starts to steam to encourage the starches to release and make it creamy, and also to stop it catching. Cook for 4–5 minutes like this, then divide between two bowls.

Make a little well in the centre and divide the strawberry compote between them, drizzling the juices over the porridge (or you can stir the compote through to make pink porridge).

Top with flaked almonds and pumpkin seeds.

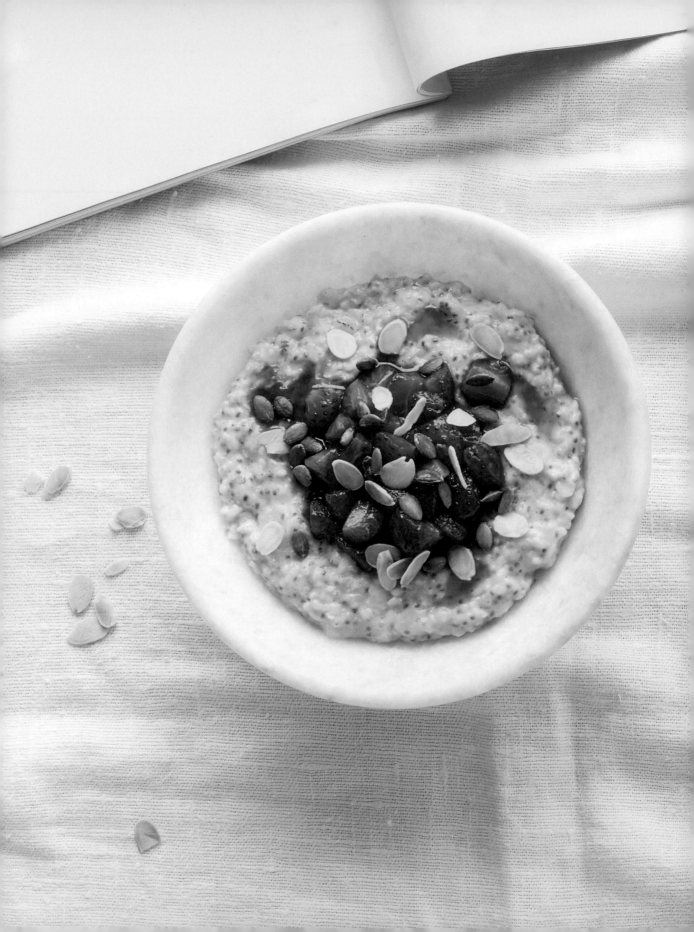

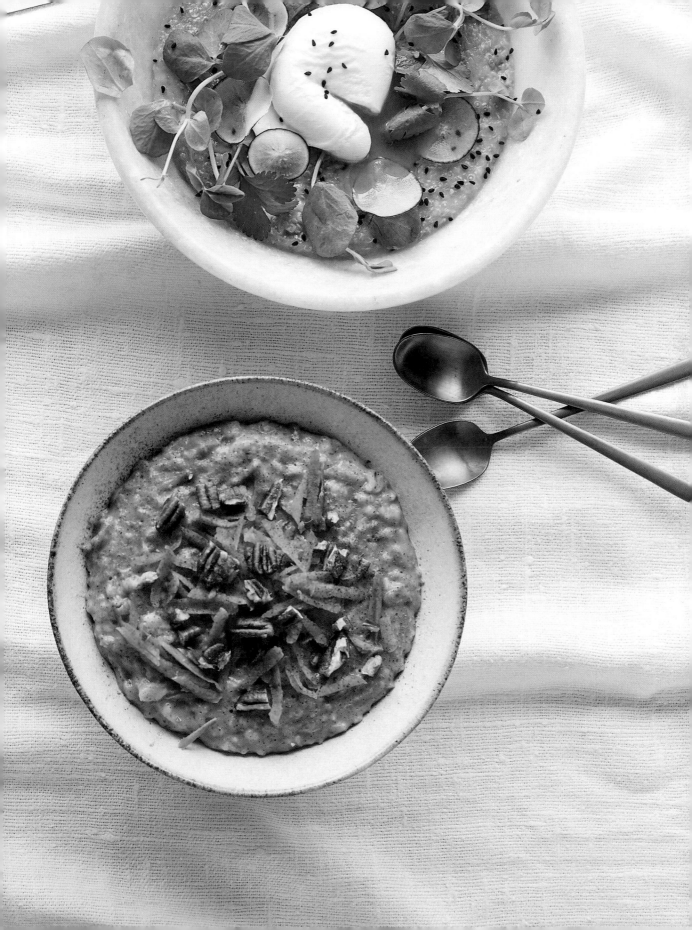

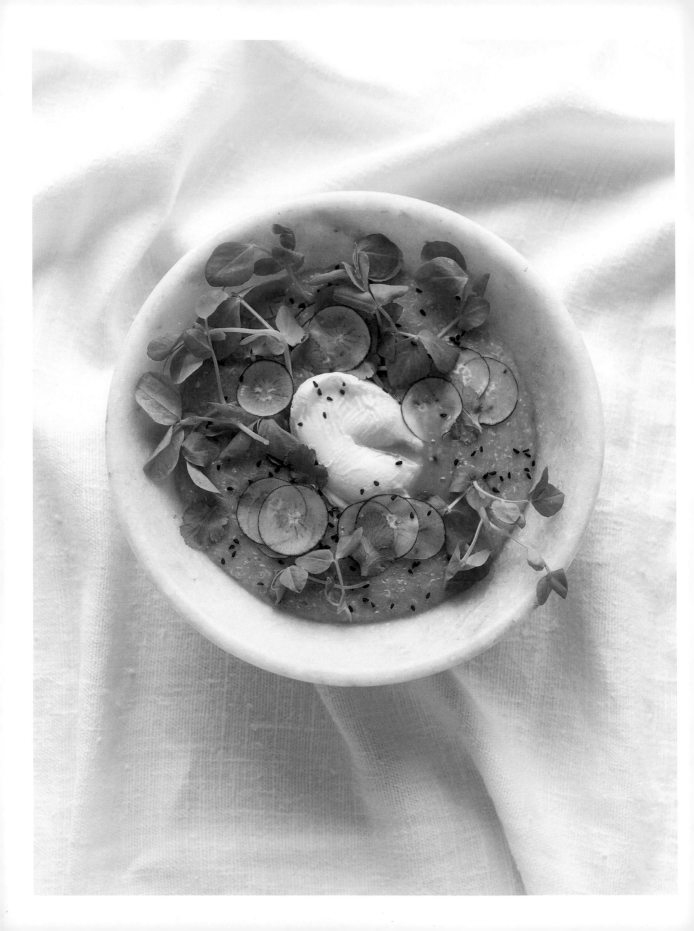

# protein porridge

serves 2

50g rolled oats

50g quinoa

600ml water

2 tbsp red miso

a splash of white wine vinegar
(optional)

2 large eggs

### for the topping

20g pea shoots

2 radishes, thinly sliced

1 tbsp coriander leaves

1 tsp nigella seeds

Add the oats, quinoa and water to a saucepan, place on a medium–low heat and cook gently for around 10–12 minutes, until the quinoa is just cooked through and the water largely absorbed.

Turn the heat right down and stir through the miso. Keep on a low heat while you poach the eggs. Bring a large saucepan of water up to simmering point. Add a splash of white wine vinegar if you have it. Crack the eggs into separate cups or ramekins. Swirl the water and then carefully tip one egg, followed by the other, into the hot water to the side of the pan. Reduce the heat to a gentle simmer and poach for 3 minutes for soft eggs, then remove with a slotted spoon and drain on kitchen paper.

Divide the porridge between two bowls and top with the pea shoots. Lay a poached egg on top and scatter over the radish slices, coriander leaves and nigella seeds. Eat straight away!

# carrot, cinnamon & pecan porridge

serves 2

75g rolled oats

25g barley flakes

1 large carrot, peeled and grated

1–2 tsp ground cinnamon, to taste,
plus extra to finish

200ml almond milk

300ml water

### for the topping

20g grated carrot

20g pecans, crumbled

Add the oats, barley flakes, grated carrot and cinnamon to a small saucepan, along with the almond milk and water. Place the pan on a medium–low heat.

Stir the porridge regularly once it starts to steam, to encourage the starches to release and make it creamy, and also to stop anything catching. Let it cook for 4–5 minutes like this. Divide between two bowls and top the porridge with the grated carrot, crumbled pecans and a little extra dusting of cinnamon.

(See previous page for photograph.)

# quick rainbow omelette with fresh salsa

I love using leftover ingredients from the fridge in my omelettes. Eggs go so well with vegetables and it is the perfect way to get your daily dose of veggies as well as a quick protein fix. I find that an omelette fills me up quicker than the same number of eggs cooked using other methods. I sometimes crumble or grate over a little cheese if I have any lying around in the fridge – Parmesan, feta or goat's cheese are all tasty options, and being full on flavour, a little goes a long way.

## serves 1

1 tsp olive oil
½ red onion, chopped
¼ red pepper, sliced
3 Tenderstem broccoli stems
30g spinach leaves
1 tsp chopped coriander
2 large eggs
salt and black pepper
1 slice of sourdough bread, toasted, to serve (optional)

### for the quick salsa

4 cherry tomatoes, roughly chopped
1 green chilli, roughly chopped
1 spring onion, roughly chopped
juice of ½ lime

Heat the olive oil in a medium frying pan and add the onion, pepper and broccoli. Gently cook for 3–4 minutes, stirring occasionally.

Add the spinach leaves and coriander and cook for another 1–2 minutes until the spinach has wilted. Remove the veg from the frying pan and keep to one side.

Assemble the salsa by simply mixing together all the ingredients in a little bowl and adding some seasoning. Keep to one side.

Whisk the eggs in a jug, tip into the frying pan and swirl around to cover the base. Add the veggies back in, arrange them evenly and season to taste.

Once the egg is cooked through, which should take a couple of minutes, slide the open omelette onto your plate and top with the salsa. Serve alongside a slice of sourdough toast, if you like.

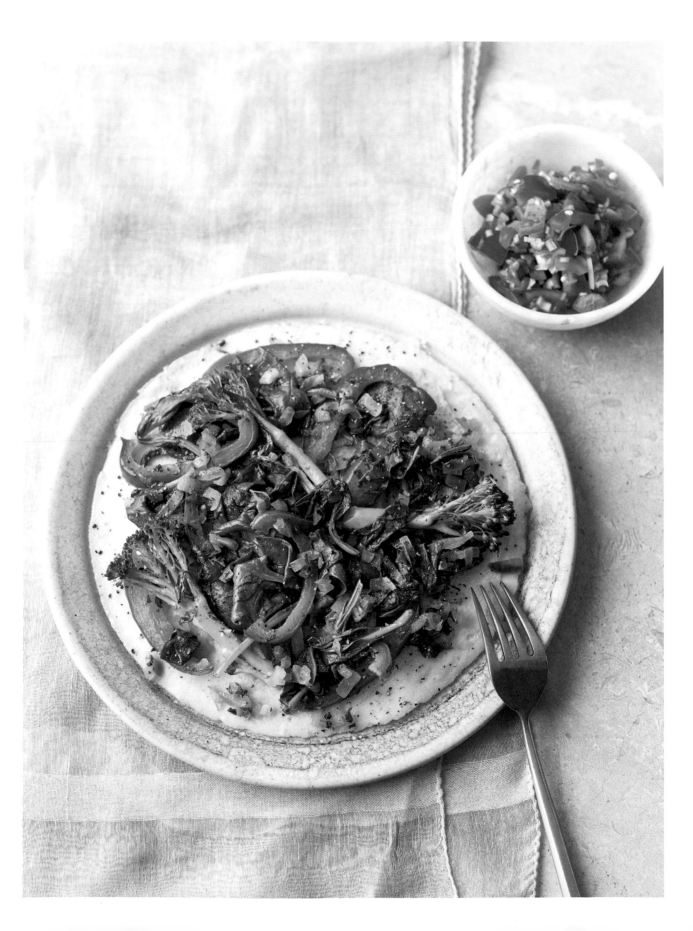

# matcha & chia seed overnight pudding

The idea of having pudding for breakfast is very appealing, and the best thing about this pud is unlike other sweet treats, it has minimal sugar, whilst boasting a great source of fibre and vegetarian protein. This recipe is super easy to make the night before, and if you make it in a jar with a lid you can even pack it up and take it with you to work! You can even turn it into a chocolate pudding by adding vanilla extract and cocoa powder; ideal to serve at a dinner party.

**serves 1**

3 tbsp chia seeds
3 tbsp oats
1 tsp matcha powder
1 tbsp fat-free Greek yoghurt
1 tbsp runny honey
250ml almond milk

In a large airtight container combine the chia seeds, oats and matcha powder. Add the yoghurt, honey and milk and stir well to combine. Put the lid on the container and place it in the fridge overnight.

> ⟨ TIP ⟩
> **I love to eat this with lots of colourful chopped fresh fruit.**

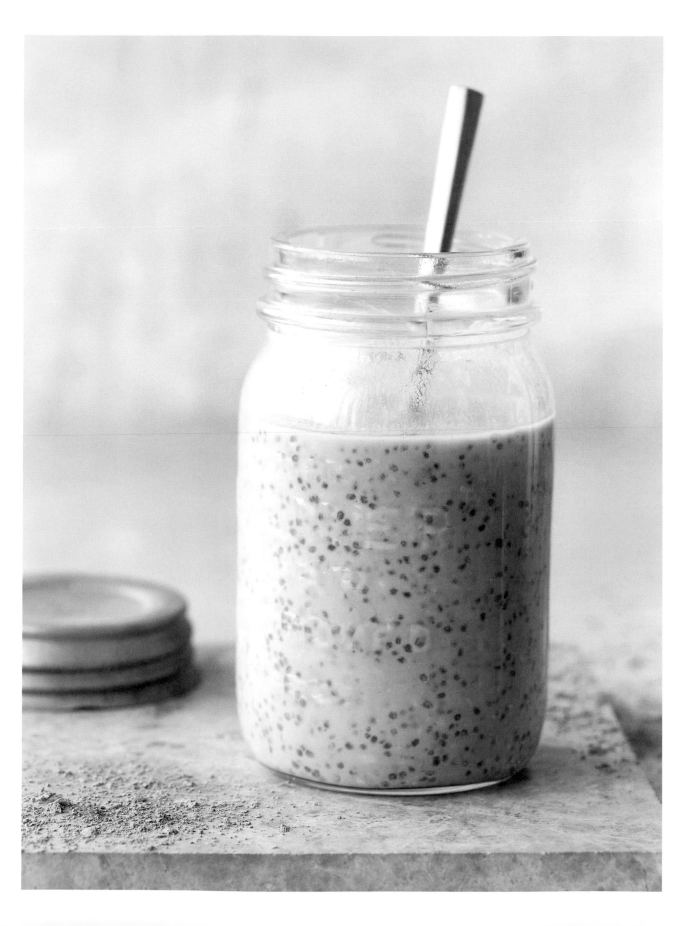

# sweet potato 'toasts' with easy toppings

I'm ALL ABOUT using vegetables to replace other ingredients, and these are the best things since sliced bread! They are my fave new discovery – the perfect breakfast base that works with both sweet and savoury toppings and equally delicious served warm or cold. *(See next page for photograph.)*

**serves 1**

2 slices of sweet potato, 5mm thick
½ tsp olive oil
salt and black pepper

Preheat your oven to 220°C/200°C fan/gas 7 and line a baking sheet with non-stick baking paper.

Brush the sweet potato slices on both sides with the olive oil and place on the baking sheet. Pop into the oven for 10 minutes, then turn the toasts over and return to the oven for a further 10 minutes.

## smashed peas & broad beans with feta and mint

80g garden peas (fresh or frozen)
50g baby broad beans
2 tsp low-fat crème fraîche
finely grated zest and juice of
   ½ lemon
20g baby spinach leaves
20g feta
1 tsp extra virgin olive oil
a few mint leaves

While the sweet potato slices are cooking, bring a saucepan of water to the boil and add the peas and broad beans. Cook for 3 minutes (or 4 for frozen), then drain into a colander. Pop the broad beans out of their skins.

Place half the peas and beans back in the saucepan and use a potato masher to crush them into a rough paste. Add the crème fraîche, lemon zest and juice and mix well. Stir through the remaining peas and beans. Keep to one side.

Once the sweet potato toast is done, transfer to a plate. Top with the baby spinach leaves and then the smashed peas and beans mixture. Crumble over the feta and drizzle over the extra virgin olive oil. Top everything with a few mint leaves and a good twist of black pepper.

## wilted spinach, roast tomato & ricotta with basil oil

1 stem of cherry tomatoes on the
  vine (about 8–10)
5g butter
100g spinach leaves
freshly grated nutmeg, to taste
1 tbsp extra virgin olive oil
1 tbsp roughly chopped basil, plus
  a few extra leaves to serve
30g ricotta

Add the stem of cherry tomatoes to the baking sheet next to the sweet potato slices for the last 10 minutes of cooking, when you turn the slices over.

Meanwhile, heat the butter in a large saucepan. Once it has melted, add the spinach and stir over a high heat until it has wilted. This will probably only take a minute or two. Squeeze any excess water from the spinach using the back of a spoon and tip it out of the pan. Grate in a little fresh nutmeg and then set aside to keep warm.

Add the extra virgin olive oil and basil to a pestle and mortar and crush the basil to make a lovely basil oil.

Remove the sweet potato toasts from the oven and spread over the ricotta. Top this with the wilted spinach and cherry tomatoes. Drizzle over the basil oil and finish off with a few extra basil leaves and a little seasoning.

## avocado, smoked salmon, cucumber, poached egg, dill

a splash of white wine vinegar
  (optional)
1 large egg
6 slices of cucumber
¼ avocado, thinly sliced
30g smoked salmon
a few sprigs of dill

While the sweet potato toasts are baking, bring a saucepan of water up to simmering point. Add a splash of white wine vinegar if you have it. Crack the egg into a small cup or ramekin. Swirl the water and then carefully tip the egg into the water to the side of the pan. Reduce to a gentle simmer and poach for 3 minutes for a soft egg, then remove with a slotted spoon and drain on kitchen paper.

Once the sweet potato toast is done, remove from the oven and put onto your serving plate, side by side. Top each with half the cucumber slices and avocado. Arrange the salmon over this and top with the poached egg. Sprinkle over some dill and season to taste.

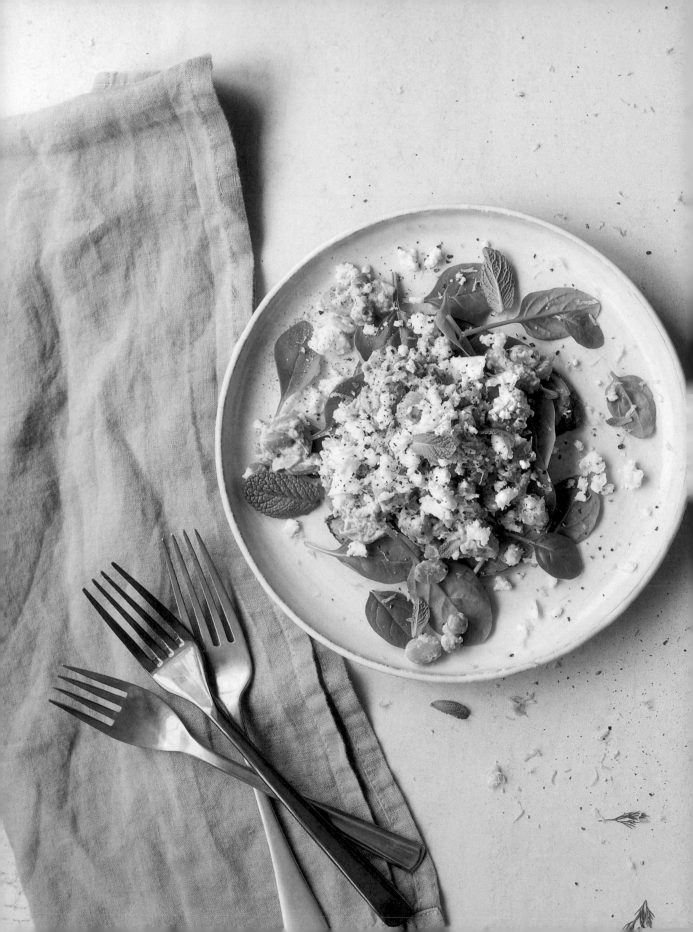

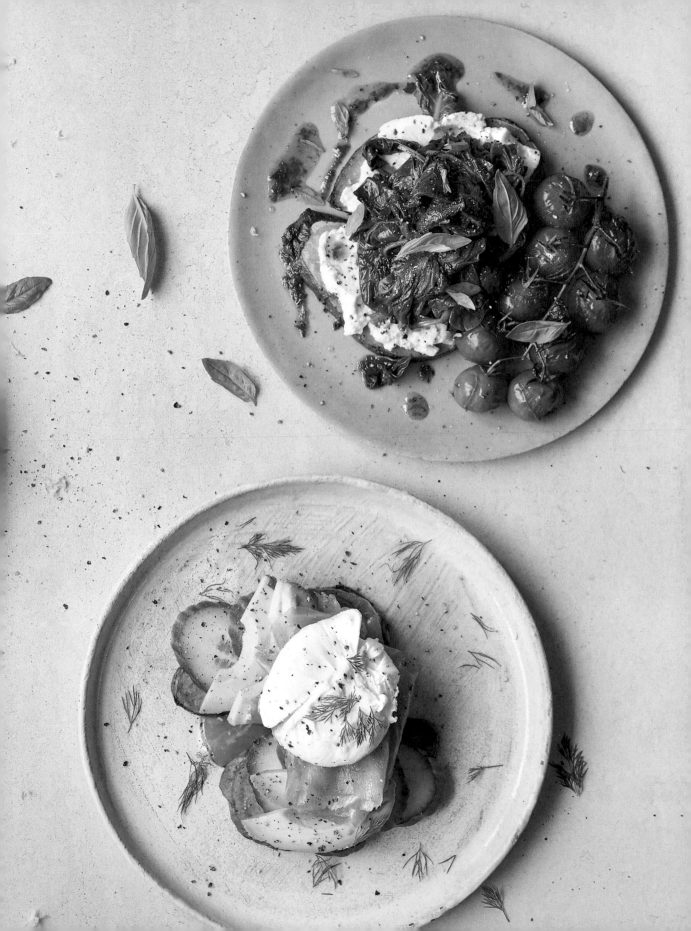

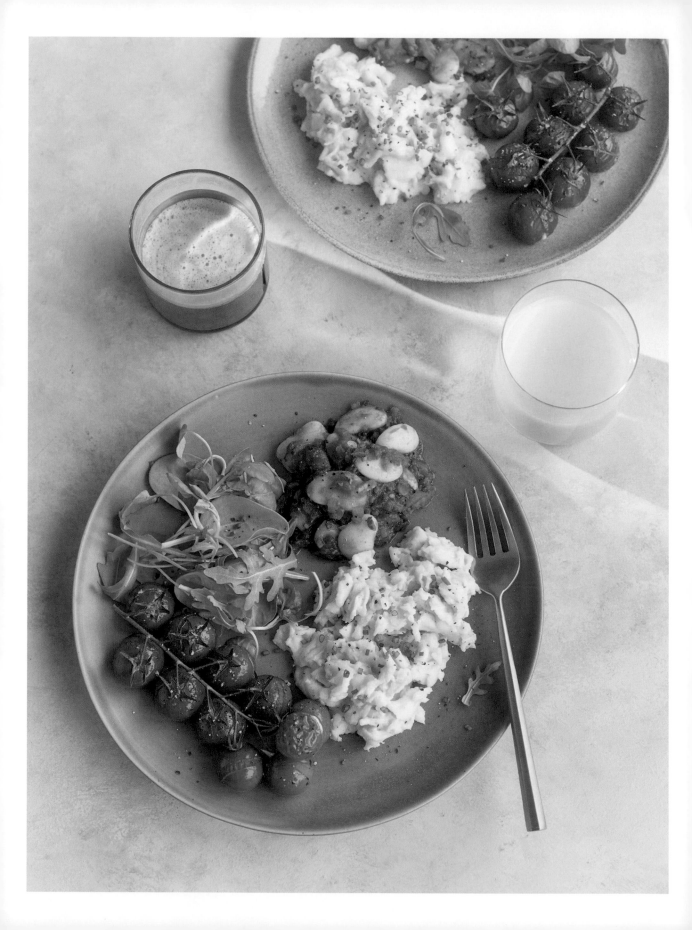

# scrambled eggs with roasted herby tomatoes, green leaves & home-made beans

I love beans because they are cheap and cheerful PLUS they contain protein, fibre and several vitamins and minerals. The beans in this recipe make enough for four servings – it will keep in the fridge for a couple of days. I like to eat them warmed up on a slice of sourdough toast for a quick post-workout snack.

## serves 2

2 sprigs of rosemary
2 stems of cherry tomatoes on the vine (about 20)
5g unsalted butter
4 medium eggs
40g green leaves
salt and black pepper
a small handful of chives, finely chopped, to serve

### for the home-made beans
### (this makes enough for
### 4 servings)
1 tsp olive oil
1 small onion, chopped
1 garlic clove, finely grated
1 x 400g tin chopped tomatoes
1 tbsp red wine vinegar
1 x 400g tin butter beans (or haricot beans), drained
1 tbsp chopped parsley

Preheat the oven to 200°C/180°C fan/gas 6 and line a baking tray with non-stick baking paper.

While the oven is warming up is the perfect time to start the beans. Heat the oil in a saucepan and add the onion. Cook for 3 minutes to start it softening and then add the garlic. Cook for another minute. Add the chopped tomatoes and vinegar and reduce the heat to a simmer. Cook for 5 minutes.

Put the rosemary sprigs onto the lined tray and place the stems of cherry tomatoes on top. Season with salt and pepper and bake in the oven for 15 minutes.

Add the butter beans to the saucepan, along with the parsley and some seasoning. Continue to cook while you finish the rest, so that the sauce thickens and reduces.

Heat the butter in a non-stick pan. While it's melting, crack the eggs into a jug and beat well. Add the eggs to the hot pan and scramble them to your liking.

Serve the scrambled egg alongside the cherry tomatoes, green leaves and some of the home-made beans. Sprinkle over some chopped chives and get stuck in.

# mixed grain breakfast platter

GOOD FOR
**post-workout**

This is a real powerhouse of a breakfast, the kind of meal I eat before a long day of filming. It has everything I need to keep me fuelled all day. It is substantial enough to work for lunch or dinner.

**serves 2**

150g butternut squash, cut into
    5mm slices
1½ tbsp olive oil
1 x 400g tin chickpeas, drained
1 tsp smoked paprika
½ tsp cayenne pepper
½ tsp ground turmeric
80g quick-cook mixed grains
    (including spelt, barley, oats etc.)
a splash of white wine vinegar
2 medium eggs
60g spinach leaves
juice of 1 lemon
40g fat-free Greek yoghurt
salt and black pepper

**to serve**
1 tsp chilli oil
1 tsp dried chilli flakes
a few sprigs of dill
lemon wedges

Preheat your oven to 220°C/200°C fan/gas 7 and line two roasting tins with non-stick baking paper.

Lay the butternut squash slices in one of the tins and drizzle over ½ tablespoon of the olive oil. Use your hands or a brush to make sure the butternut is well covered. Season with a little salt and pepper.

Add the chickpeas to the other roasting tin and drizzle over the remaining tablespoon of oil. Sprinkle over the paprika, cayenne and turmeric. Shake the tray to coat the chickpeas evenly in the spices. Pop both roasting tins into the oven and roast for 25 minutes, turning the squash and shaking both trays halfway through the cooking time.

While they are roasting, place the grains in a saucepan and rinse well under running water. Drain, cover with cold water and bring to the boil, then reduce to a simmer and cook for around 12 minutes.

Bring a saucepan of water up to simmering point. Add a splash of white wine vinegar if you have it. Crack the eggs into separate cups or ramekins. Swirl the water and then carefully tip one egg, followed by the other, into the water, to the side of the pan. Reduce to a gentle simmer and poach for 3 minutes for soft eggs, then remove with a slotted spoon and drain on kitchen paper.

Once the grains are cooked, drain and return them to the saucepan. Add the spinach leaves, lemon juice and lots of seasoning and stir the leaves through to wilt in the heat of the grains.

Spread the grains out on a serving dish and top with the squash slices. Dollop with the yoghurt and top with the eggs. Add half the crispy chickpeas (save the rest to snack on). Drizzle over the chilli oil and sprinkle over the chilli flakes and fresh dill. Serve with lemon wedges.

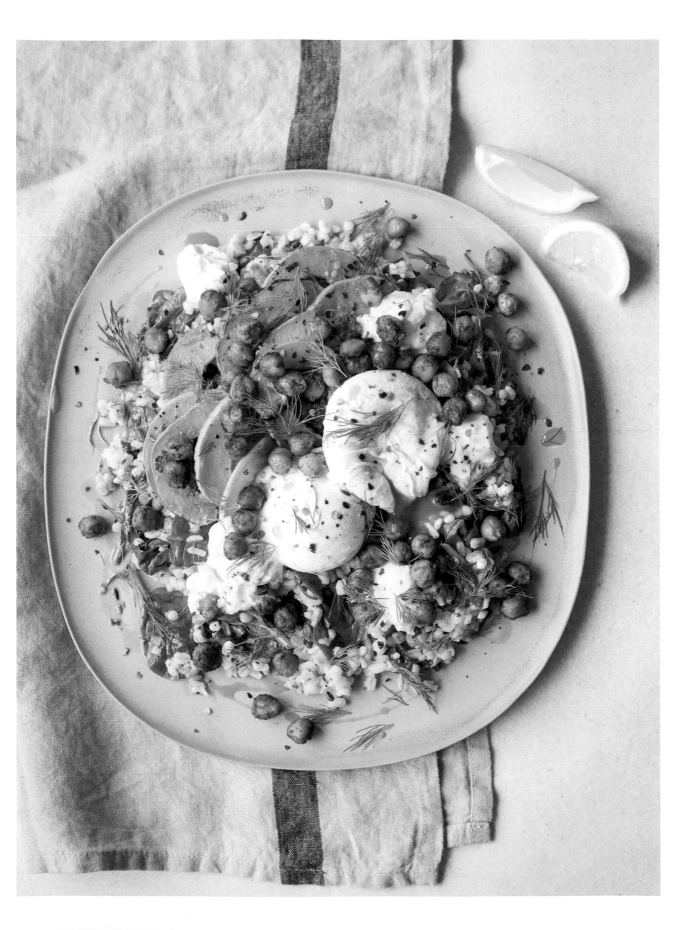

# breakfast stir-fry

Our culture has developed a pretty strong idea of what constitutes breakfast but don't be put off by the idea of a more savoury option. It's a great way to get a head start on healthy eating at the beginning of the day.

## serves 2

2 x 125g salmon fillets, skin on

2 tsp toasted sesame oil

4 spring onions, sliced

1 red chilli, finely chopped

1 garlic clove, thinly sliced

1 tbsp roughly chopped coriander, plus extra leaves to serve

100g shiitake mushrooms, sliced

80g spring greens, sliced into ribbons

1 tbsp low-salt soy sauce

2 tsp mirin

1 tsp rice wine vinegar

toasted sesame seeds, to serve

Preheat your grill to its highest setting and place the salmon, skin side up, on a baking tray that will fit under it. Cook for 4 minutes and then flip the fillets over and cook for another 4 minutes. Keep to one side until you need them.

Heat the sesame oil in a large wok over a medium heat and add the spring onions, chilli, garlic and coriander. Cook for 2 minutes, stirring often so nothing sticks and burns. Add the mushrooms and spring greens and increase the heat, tossing and flicking the pan to keep everything moving and cooking evenly. It should only take about 3 minutes for everything to be cooked.

Add the soy, mirin and rice wine vinegar.

Take the salmon fillets and use the back of a fork to press down on the top to break them into lovely big flakes. Divide the mushrooms and spring greens between two plates and top with the salmon flakes. Add some sesame seeds and fresh coriander and serve immediately.

⟨ TIP ⟩
**Also great topped with a poached egg each instead of the salmon.**

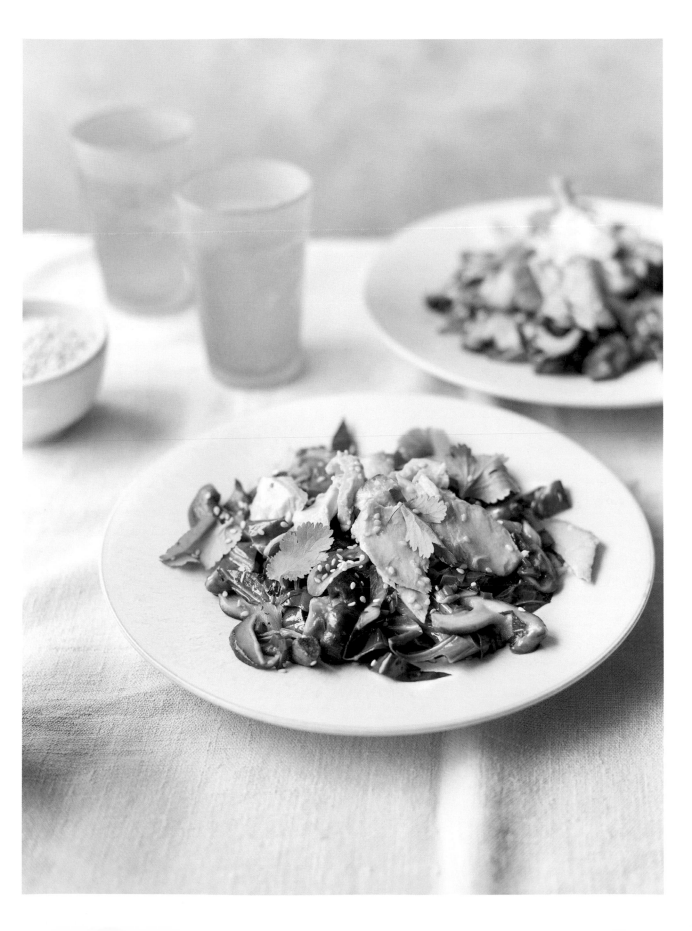

# turkish eggs & halloumi

I love the silkiness of the poached eggs against the sour yoghurt with a fresh kick from the parsley. This is a tasty option that I like to treat my friends or family to on the weekend.

## serves 2

4 slices of halloumi, about 5mm thick

1 tsp olive oil

½ tsp ground turmeric

½ tsp freshly ground black pepper, plus extra to serve

140g Greek yoghurt

1 garlic clove, finely grated

1 tbsp extra virgin olive oil

1 tbsp dried chilli flakes, plus extra to serve

a splash of white wine vinegar (optional)

2 medium eggs

a good handful each of dill and parsley, roughly chopped

salt

Preheat the oven to 200°C/180°C fan/gas 6.

Line a roasting tin with non-stick baking paper and lay out the halloumi slices. Sprinkle the olive oil, turmeric and black pepper over the halloumi and then turn the slices in the mix to make sure they are well coated.

Pop the tray into the hot oven to bake for 10–12 minutes until golden brown around the edges.

Meanwhile, whisk together the Greek yoghurt, garlic, extra virgin olive oil and chilli flakes in a mixing bowl.

Bring a large saucepan of water up to simmering point. Add a splash of white wine vinegar if you have it. Crack the eggs into separate cups or ramekins. Swirl the water and then carefully tip one egg, followed by the other, into the hot water, to the side of the pan. Reduce to a gentle simmer and poach for 3 minutes for soft eggs, then remove with a slotted spoon and drain on kitchen paper.

Add the eggs to the yoghurt mix, carefully coating them.

Divide the halloumi between two plates and top each with a yoghurt-coated egg.

Scatter over lots and lots of the fresh herbs, an extra sprinkle of chilli flakes, and salt and pepper to taste.

〈 TIP 〉
**Instead of halloumi you could serve this on sweet potato toasts.**

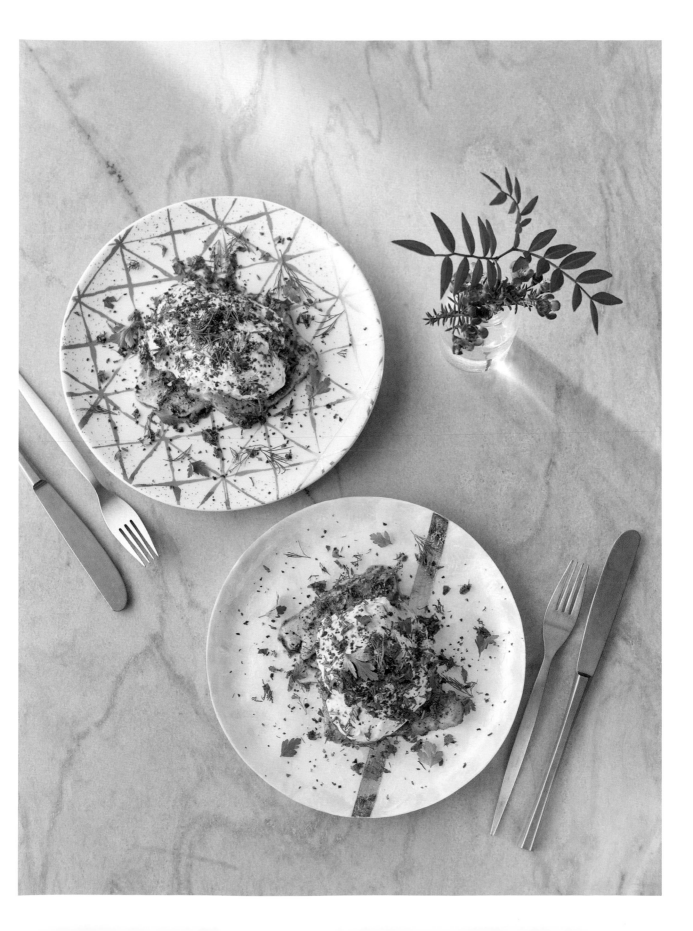

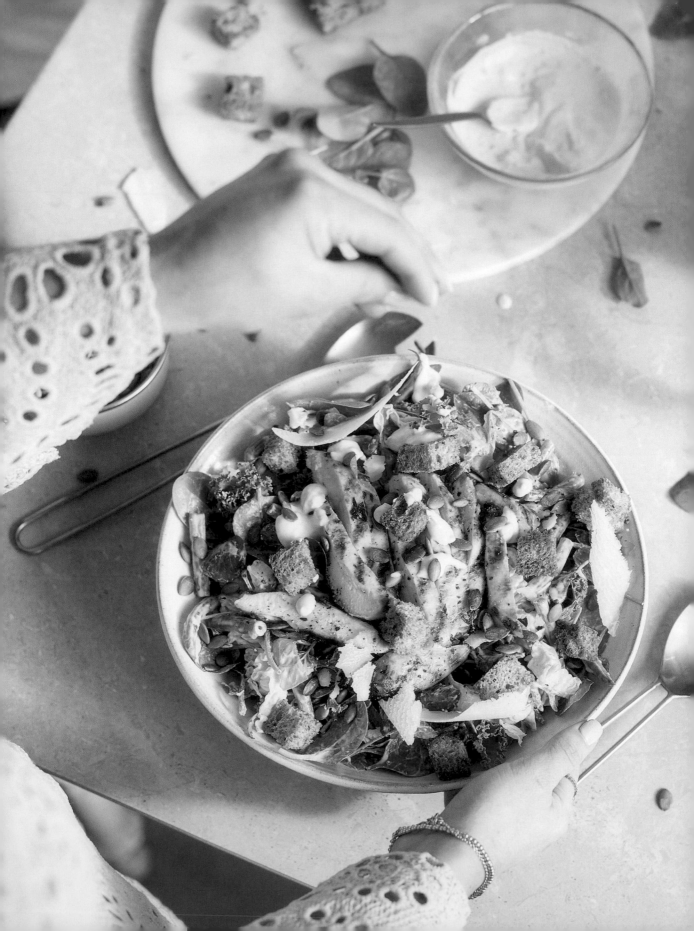

lunch

# mozzarella salad with broad beans, peas, mint & a lemony dressing

This is the dreamiest of salad recipes to get familiar with because it can be thrown together for multiple purposes. It works PERFECTLY as a lunch for when I'm craving something light and fresh or if I know I have a dinner party to go to in the evening and I'm likely to be well fed. I also serve it as a large sharing dish to accompany a main course.

## serves 2 as a main

125g mozzarella ball
120g peas (fresh or frozen)
100g broad beans (fresh or frozen)
60g pomegranate seeds
2 tbsp shredded mint leaves
100g pea shoots
juice of 1 lemon
2 tbsp extra virgin olive oil
salt and black pepper

< TIP >
**For a more filling meal, serve this alongside some simply cooked chicken.**

Drain the mozzarella and leave to one side to come up to room temperature (it's more delicious when it's not fridge-cold because it softens a bit).

Bring a pan of water to the boil and add the peas and broad beans. Bring back to the boil then cook for about 3 minutes for fresh, 4 minutes for frozen; you want them to still have some crunch to them. Drain into a colander and run under cold water until they no longer feel warm to the touch.

Remove the outer skins from the broad beans to reveal the sweet, bright green bean inside. Give the peas and beans a good shake to remove any excess water.

Add the pomegranate seeds, mint and pea shoots to a mixing bowl. Tear the mozzarella ball roughly into 8 pieces and add to the bowl then toss everything together. Transfer to a serving plate and top with the peas and beans.

Put the lemon juice and extra virgin olive oil in a small bowl (or clean jam jar). Season to taste, mix well and give it a quick taste to check it's the right balance of acidity for you. If you like it sharper, just add a few more drops of lemon juice.

Drizzle a little dressing over the salad and serve the rest on the side.

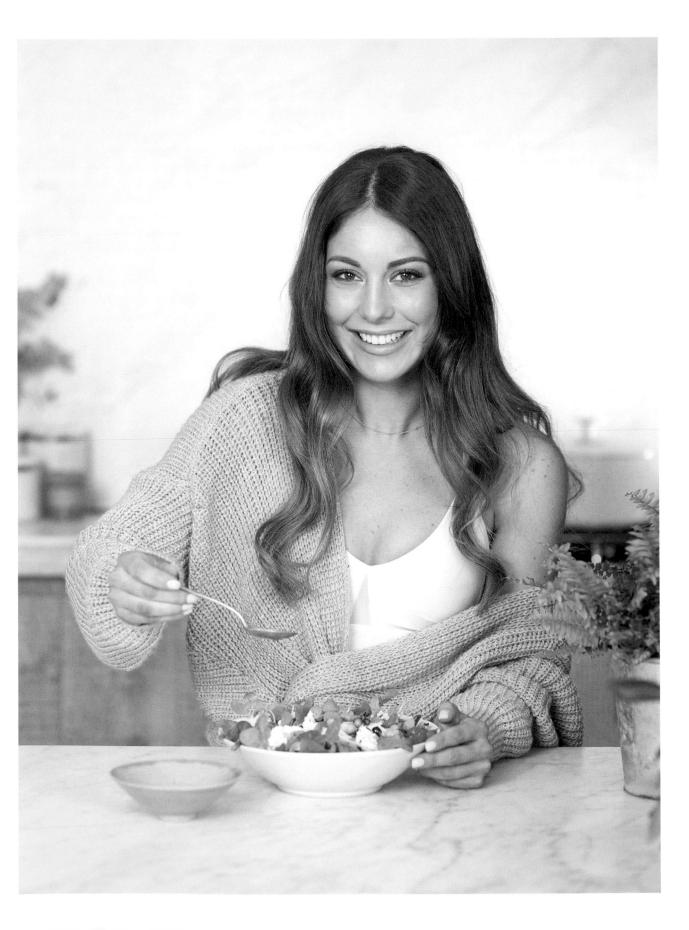

# tuna, mango & avocado salad

This salad puts a smile across my face. I'm aware that fresh tuna and mango tend to be expensive ingredients so I prepare this on special occasions when I need a pick-me-up or if I'm trying to impress someone.

## serves 2

2 x 120g tuna steaks

1 tsp olive oil

1 tbsp mixed sesame seeds, plus extra to serve

60g mixed green leaves

2 spring onions, sliced

1 red chilli, halved, deseeded and thinly sliced

1 mango, sliced

½ avocado, sliced

1 nori sheet

### for the dressing

2 tbsp lemon juice

2 tbsp extra-virgin olive oil

¼ tsp wasabi, or more to taste

finely grated zest and juice of 1 lime

Place the tuna on a chopping board and brush the olive oil all over the steaks. Place the sesame seeds in a shallow bowl and roll the side edges of the steaks in the seeds.

Heat a frying pan on a high heat and add the tuna. Cook for 90 seconds then flip and cook the other side for 90 seconds. Then very carefully, using a pair of tongs, slowly roll the sesame seed-coated edges in the hot pan to fully sear the fish. This will keep it pink in the middle, but you can cook it for longer if you'd rather it cooked through. Remove from the heat and leave to rest and cool.

In a small bowl, whisk together the dressing ingredients and set aside.

Divide the mixed green leaves between your serving plates. Add the spring onions, chilli, mango and avocado to the serving plates. Drizzle the dressing over the salad. Slice the tuna steak into thin slices and top the salad with it. Crumble over the nori sheet and add an extra sprinkling of sesame seeds.

⟨ TIP ⟩
**Make sure your mangos are lovely and ripe!**

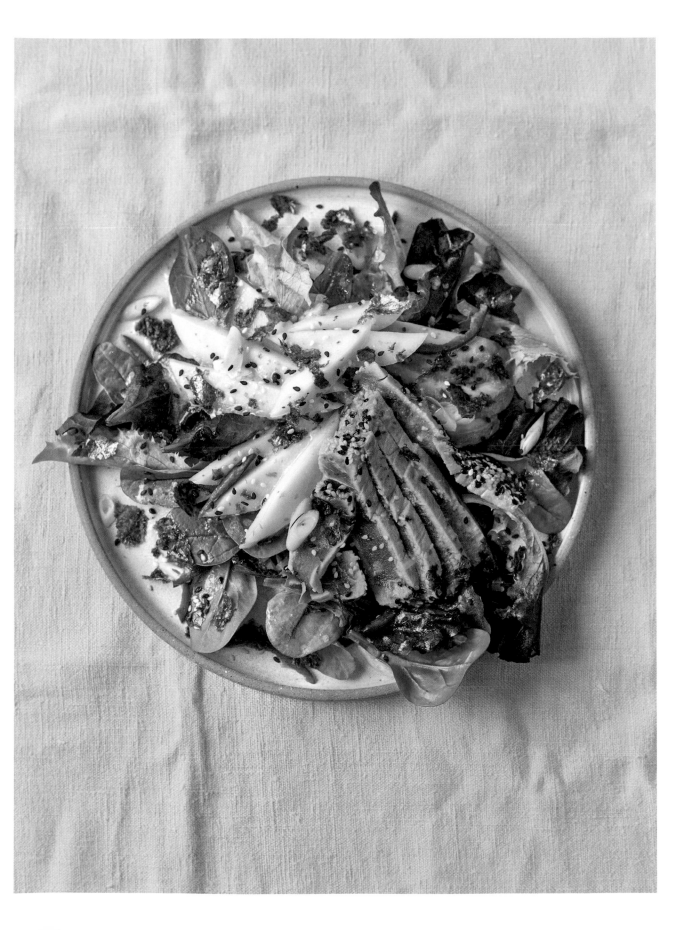

# chicken caesar salad

GOOD FOR
*post-*
workout

I like to scale up this recipe for when I have people round for a relaxed lunch. I serve it in a large bowl that my mum gifted me and let people help themselves.

## serves 2

1 large boneless, skinless chicken
   breast
1 tsp olive oil
1 small garlic clove, crushed
juice of ½ lemon
a sprig of fresh thyme, leaves only
   (use dried if you don't have fresh)
80g green beans, trimmed
½ Romaine lettuce, or 1 baby gem
   lettuce, washed and sliced
30g salad leaves (to include
   watercress, spinach and rocket)
30g kale, leaves torn and tough
   stalks removed
15g Parmesan shavings

### for the croûtons
2 medium slices of wholemeal bread
   (about 60g in total)
1 tbsp pumpkin seeds
1 tbsp olive oil
salt and black pepper

### for the dressing
1½ tbsp lemon juice
3 anchovies in oil, finely chopped
   (I know a lot of people don't like
   anchovies but they add a nice salty
   flavour; if you have an aversion just
   omit them)
¾ tsp Worcestershire sauce
4 tbsp fat-free Greek yoghurt
½ tsp wholegrain mustard
½ tsp Dijon mustard
1 small garlic clove, crushed

Preheat your oven to 200°C/180°C fan/gas 6.

Place the chicken breast on a sheet of baking paper and fold the paper over the top. Take a rolling pin and give it a quick bash to even out the thickness to around 1cm (this tenderises it and makes it quicker to cook). Place in a dish with the olive oil, garlic, lemon juice and thyme. Set aside for 10 minutes to marinate.

Cut the bread for the croûtons into 1.5cm cubes and place on a baking sheet along with the pumpkin seeds. Drizzle over the olive oil and season well. Place in the hot oven for 8 minutes, then remove, turn and return for another 5–8 minutes until golden brown and crisp.

Bring a pan of water to the boil and blanch the green beans for 4 minutes, so they still have some crunch to them, then drain and rinse under cold running water to cool them slightly. Once you can handle them, cut each bean into three and add to a mixing bowl.

Heat a griddle pan over a high heat and shake most of the marinade off the chicken. When the griddle is hot, add the chicken and cook for 6 minutes, then turn and cook for another 6 minutes (or until it's cooked through). Move to a chopping board to rest.

Make the dressing by whisking all the ingredients together in a small bowl.

Add all salad leaves and kale to the mixing bowl with the beans. Add half the dressing and toss everything together to coat the leaves and beans. Transfer to a serving dish; slice the chicken breast into strips and place over the leaves. Drizzle the rest of the dressing over the salad and top with the croûtons and pumpkin seeds.

Add the Parmesan shavings and serve.

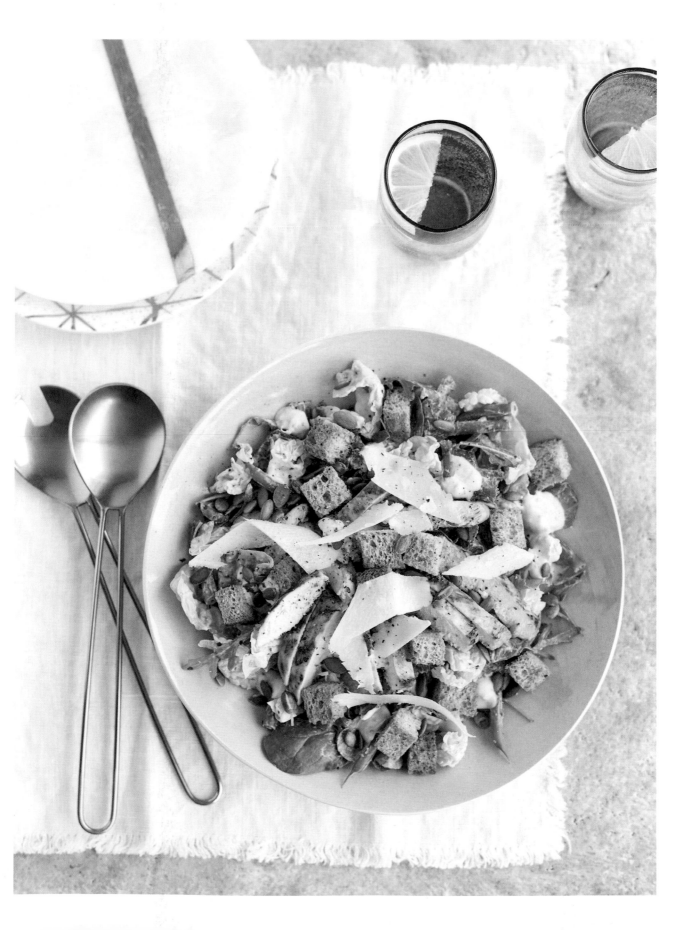

# halloumi salad with spinach, red onion, pomegranate and balsamic

**pack up & go** OPTION

Balsamic and red onion is a match made in heaven.
If you have a bit of extra time, wilt the red onions in a pan
slowly in a little oil for around 20 minutes and when soft add the
balsamic and a sprinkle of sugar to caramelise.

### serves 2

4 slices of halloumi, about 5mm thick
½ tsp olive oil
40g baby spinach leaves
40g rocket leaves
½ red onion, thinly sliced
40g pomegranate seeds
2 tsp roughly chopped parsley
balsamic vinegar, to drizzle
2 tsp runny honey
black pepper
20g walnuts, toasted and roughly
   chopped, to serve

Brush the halloumi slices with the olive oil, season with black pepper and heat a frying pan on a high heat. Add the halloumi to the pan and cook for 2 minutes on each side, or until golden brown. Then remove from the pan and allow to cool a little while you make the rest of the salad.

Add the spinach, rocket, red onion, pomegranate seeds and parsley to a large mixing bowl and gently mix everything together. Drizzle over the balsamic vinegar and honey and season to taste with black pepper; toss to coat everything.

Divide the salad between two serving bowls. Cut each halloumi slice into two strips and place on top of the salad.

Crumble over the walnuts and enjoy.

〈 TIP 〉
**This easy dressing is great on all kinds of salad.**

# salmon parcels with quinoa & a parsley–lemon dressing

I cook salmon at least once a week because I know that it is a solid source of omega 3 and good fats (great for hair, skin and nails). There is an abundance of quick and tasty ways to cook it. I can't get enough of cooking in tin foil because then I don't have to battle with washing up at the end of my meal.

## serves 2

2 x 120g salmon fillets
6 Tenderstem broccoli tips
2 stems of cherry tomatoes on the vine (about 8–10 on each)
20g butter, softened
finely grated zest and juice of 1 lemon
1 tbsp roughly chopped parsley
80g quinoa
50g rocket leaves
salt and black pepper
lemon wedges, to serve

Preheat your oven to 200°C/180°C fan/gas 6.

Take two large pieces of tin foil and lay them on your work surface. Lay a salmon fillet in the middle of each one. Put the broccoli on each side and a stem of cherry tomatoes on top, then keep to one side.

Put the butter into a small mixing bowl and use a fork to soften it into a paste. Add the lemon zest, parsley and some salt and pepper. Use the fork to press everything into the butter.

Divide the butter in two and add to the salmon parcels, along with the lemon juice.

Bring up the sides of the foil and scrunch it together to seal it into two airtight parcels. Place the parcels on a baking sheet and pop into the hot oven for 20 minutes.

Meanwhile, cook the quinoa. Add it to a saucepan, cover with cold water, bring it up to the boil on a medium–high heat, then reduce the heat, put a lid on and simmer for around 10–12 minutes, or until cooked.

Drain the quinoa and stir in some seasoning and the rocket. Divide it between two serving plates and remove the salmon from the oven. Open the parcels up (take care as very hot steam will escape) and, using a metal spatula or fish slice, carefully lift the salmon and veg on top of the quinoa and rocket. Drizzle over the buttery juices from the foil parcels and serve with some lemon wedges.

# butternut squash soup

Few things are as comforting as a hot bowl of soup. I can get creative with what I put in them plus they are a great way of incorporating lots of nutritious vegetables into your diet. People often associate eating soup as a main meal as 'diet food', however, the more you experiment with them you'll soon realise that they can really fill you up. The roasted butternut squash and pepper add a rich flavour and consistency to this recipe.

## serves 4

1 large butternut squash, peeled, deseeded and diced

1 red pepper, deseeded and cut into chunks

2 tbsp olive oil

1 onion, chopped

2 celery sticks, chopped

2 carrots, peeled and chopped

2 garlic cloves, finely chopped

1 tbsp chopped sage

1 litre vegetable stock

salt and black pepper

4 tbsp natural yoghurt, to serve

Preheat your oven to 200°C/180°C fan/gas 6.

Put the squash and red pepper into a roasting tin, drizzle over half the olive oil and season well with salt and pepper.

Pop into the oven for 20–25 minutes until everything has started to turn golden brown around the edges and the squash has softened.

With 10 minutes to go on the squash, heat a large saucepan with the remaining oil and add the onion, celery and carrots. Cook on a low heat for 10 minutes, stirring often until everything has softened and turned lightly golden.

Add the garlic and sage and cook for another minute, then add the roasted squash and pepper straight from the oven.

Add the stock and bring to the boil, then turn down and simmer for 10 minutes. Use either a stick blender, blender or food processor to blitz everything until super smooth.

Season to taste with salt and pepper. Pour into four serving bowls and swirl 1 tablespoon of yoghurt into each, before adding your choice of topping.

< TIP >
**Soups are great to pack up and take to work**

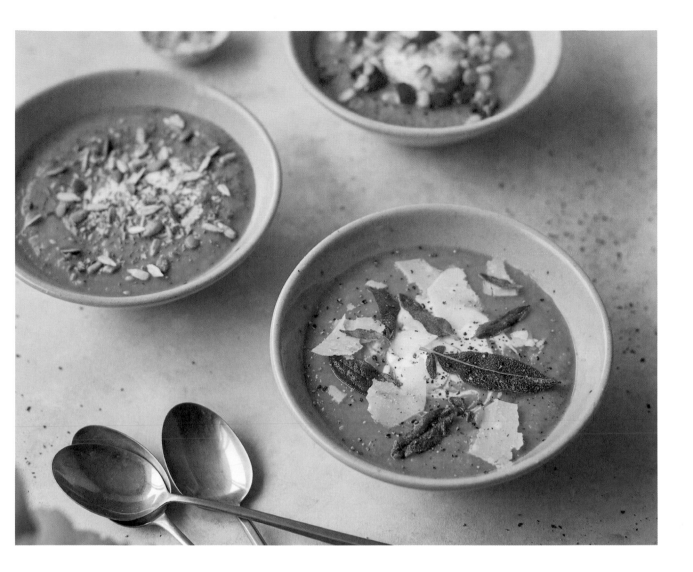

## for the toppings

These are some suggestions of quick and easy toppings for the soup – feel free to mix it up and go with what you fancy.

### seed mix

1 tbsp pumpkin seeds
1 tbsp sunflower seeds
1 tbsp milled flaxseeds
1 tbsp poppy seeds

Spread all the seeds out on a baking tray and toast in the oven for 12–15 minutes alongside the squash, until golden. Sprinkle a little handful onto your soup.

### sage leaf topping

1 tbsp olive oil
20 sage leaves
40g Parmesan shavings

Heat the oil in a small frying pan and add the sage leaves. Fry until crisp then drain on kitchen paper to remove the excess oil. Add to the soup then scatter over some Parmesan shavings.

### veg topping

1 red pepper, deseeded and diced
1 x 380g tin sweetcorn, drained
1 tbsp olive oil

Pop the pepper and corn into a small roasting tin and toss in the oil with some salt and pepper. Roast in the oven for 20 minutes alongside the squash. Top your soup with them.

# three throw-together pasta dishes

Pasta is an ideal lunch or dinner option when you're short on time. Wholewheat pasta means extra fibre and subbing butternut or courgette 'spaghetti' is a clever way of getting even more vegetables into your meals. I've paired each sauce with my favourite combination of pasta, but feel free to mix them up according to your taste buds. You can top these dishes with some rocket leaves and extra Parmesan to garnish if you like – the taste of the peppery rocket and salty cheese will add extra indulgence to these sauces. *(See next page for photograph.)*

serves 2

## avocado pesto with butternut noodles

180g cherry tomatoes, halved
1 butternut squash, peeled, halved and deseeded

### for the pesto
1 avocado, in chunks
2 tbsp torn basil, plus extra leaves to serve
1 small garlic clove, grated
2 tbsp extra virgin olive oil
20g Parmesan, finely grated, plus extra shavings to serve
salt and black pepper

Preheat the oven to 200°C/180°C fan/gas 6.

For the pesto, place the avocado in a mini-chopper or food processor with the torn basil, garlic and extra virgin olive oil. Blitz to a paste then transfer to a small bowl. Stir through the grated Parmesan and a little seasoning.

Place the cherry tomatoes cut side up on a baking sheet and pop them into the hot oven for 8–10 minutes, until you can see them softening nicely.

Bring a pan of water to the boil with a steamer basket and lid on top. While it is coming to the boil, use a spiraliser to turn the butternut squash into spaghetti noodles. Place in the steamer and cook for 3–4 minutes, or until al dente. Drain the saucepan and tip the noodles into the saucepan.

Add the pesto and toss to coat the noodles.

Divide between two bowls, top with the semi-roasted tomatoes, some basil leaves, Parmesan shavings and some seasoning, to taste.

## creamy mushroom sauce with wholewheat spagetti

GOOD FOR
post-workout

150g wholewheat spaghetti

**for the creamy mushroom sauce**

1 tsp olive oil
120g button mushrooms, sliced
1 large egg, plus 1 extra yolk
40g Parmesan, finely grated
2 tbsp chopped parsley
salt and black pepper

In a frying pan with the olive oil over a high heat, cook the mushrooms for 5 minutes, tossing the pan, until they are golden brown. Slide out of the pan and keep to one side.

Bring a large saucepan of salted water to the boil. Cook the pasta according to the packet instructions – usually around 10–12 minutes. While the pasta is cooking, place the whole egg and egg yolk in a jug and beat together with the Parmesan and some black pepper.

When the pasta is done, scoop out 2 tablespoons of the cooking water, then drain it into a colander and pop it back into the saucepan. Turn the heat on as low as it goes and scoop in the egg mixture along with the cooking water. Stir furiously to coat the pasta; don't let it get too hot as you don't want scrambled egg. It should become a silky, creamy sauce that clings to the pasta. Add the mushrooms and toss to incorporate. Stir through the parsley and divide between two dishes to serve.

## easy-peasy puttanesca with courgetti

3 courgettes, trimmed

**for the puttanesca sauce**

2 tbsp olive oil
1 red onion, diced
2 garlic cloves, thinly sliced
2 anchovies in oil, finely chopped
1 tbsp tomato purée
1 tsp dried chilli flakes
1 x 400g tin plum tomatoes
40g black olives, pitted and halved
1 tbsp capers, rinsed and chopped
a small handful of parsley leaves, roughly chopped
grated zest and juice of 1 lemon
salt and black pepper

Heat the olive oil in a large pan and add the onion, garlic and anchovies. Cook gently for about 5 minutes until everything starts to soften and the anchovies have largely broken down. Add the tomato purée and stir to mix well, allowing it to cook for a minute to let the flavours develop before adding the chilli flakes and tinned tomatoes.

Break the tomatoes open with the back of your spoon and allow the sauce to simmer and thicken gently for around 5–6 minutes. Add the olives and capers and stir to mix.

Use a spiraliser to turn the courgettes into spaghetti. Add these directly to the sauce and cook everything together for just 2 minutes. You don't want the courgette to get soft – it's much nicer while it's still a little crunchy. Take off the heat, stir through the parsley and lemon zest and squeeze over a little lemon juice. Divide between two bowls, season to taste and serve.

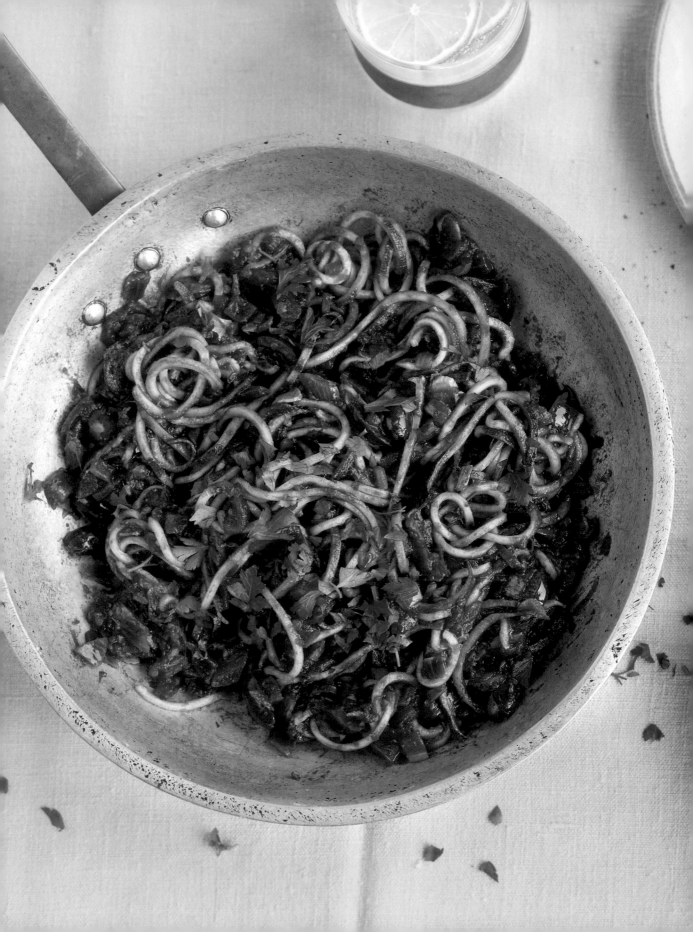

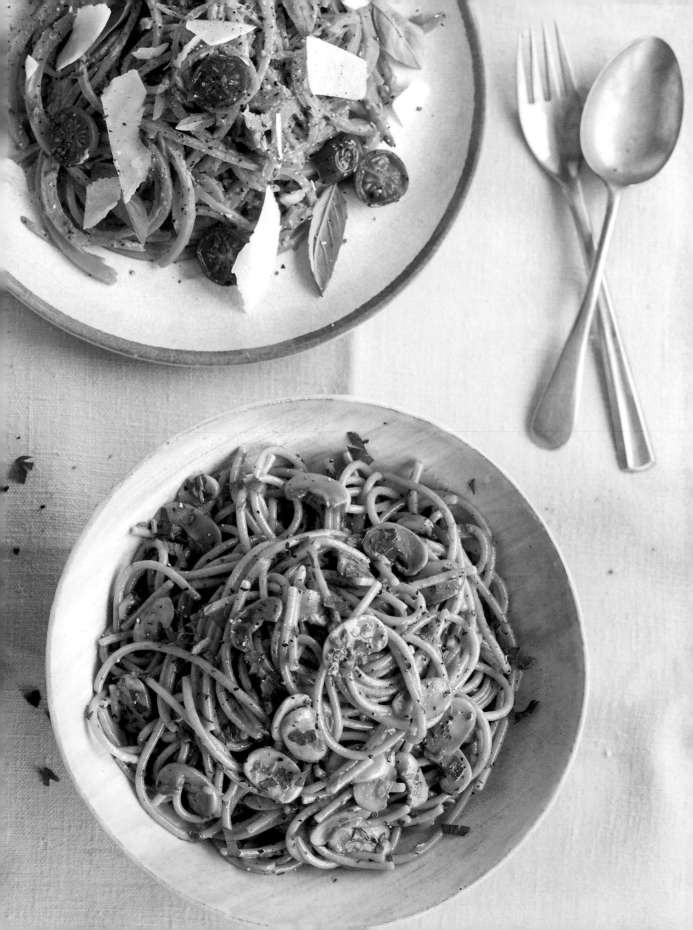

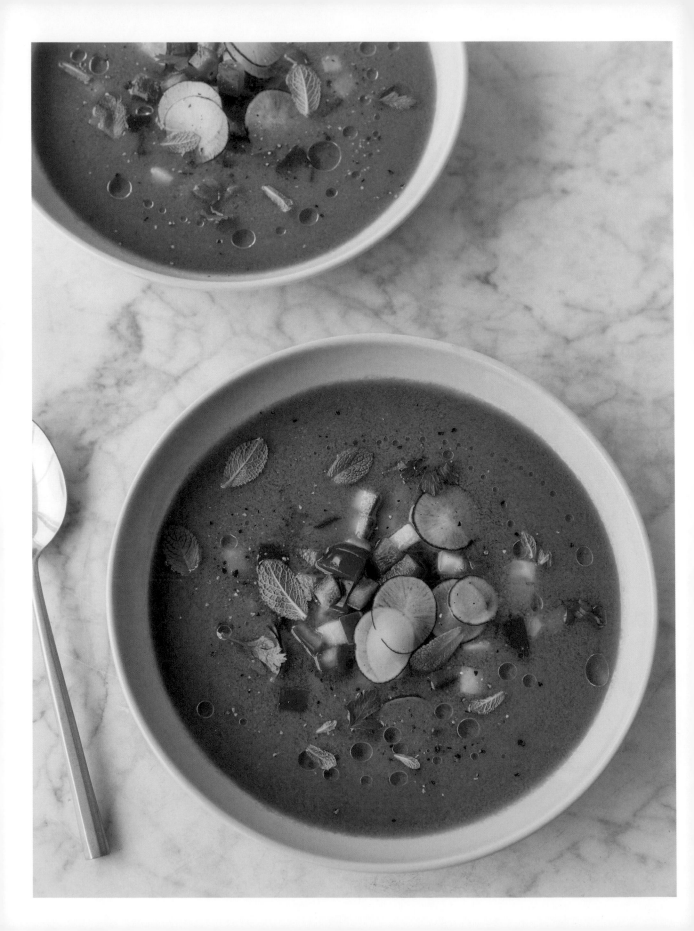

# gazpacho

pack up
& go
OPTION

I fell in love with gazpacho when I lived in Mougins, a small village in the south of France, for two months while filming for the show in the summer of 2015. I know gazpacho doesn't originate from France but it resonates there for me. It is probably the freshest thing I've ever tasted. Some people find the concept of cold soup odd but don't knock it until you've tried it. I like to add lots of diced cucumber and radish to the top to add crunch.

## serves 4

100g stale bread
1 red pepper, deseeded and
   roughly chopped
1 green pepper, deseeded and
   roughly chopped
1kg tomatoes, roughly chopped
1 cucumber, peeled, deseeded and
   roughly chopped
2 garlic cloves, crushed
about 2 tbsp extra virgin olive oil,
   plus a few drops to serve
about 2 tbsp sherry vinegar (or red
   wine vinegar)
salt and black pepper

### for the garnish options
finely sliced radishes
finely diced cucumber
finely chopped pepper
mint leaves
parsley leaves

If you are using bread (it thickens the gazpacho nicely), start by soaking it in cold water for 10 minutes.

Put the peppers, tomatoes, cucumber and garlic in a blender or food processor and blitz until very smooth. This will take a few minutes; don't forget to scrape down the sides to make sure you've got everything.

Gently squeeze out any excess moisture from the soaked bread and tear it into pieces straight into the blender or processor, before blending again until smooth.

Taste the soup then add extra virgin olive oil, vinegar and salt and pepper to taste. Give it a quick pulse to mix then pour it out into a large jug or pan through a sieve to remove any last bits. This is a bonus step because the gazpacho is much more desirable if it is VERY silky.

Drizzle over a few drops of extra virgin olive oil and serve with your choice of garnish, or a mixture of them all.

# poached chicken & spicy yoghurt lettuce boats

Whoever came up with the idea of trading a bread-based wrap with green leaves is a genius. A wrap is simply a device to contain or hold a tasty middle and it rarely serves much purpose on the taste front. These lettuce leaves add a delicious fresh crunch too.

## serves 4 as a main

2 large boneless, skinless chicken breasts, halved horizontally

1 tbsp low-salt soy sauce

100g green beans, trimmed and cut into 5cm pieces

5g unsalted butter

1 tsp olive oil

1 onion, finely chopped

juice of 2 limes

2 tbsp Greek yoghurt

2 tbsp hoisin sauce

1 bunch of spring onions, finely chopped

2 tbsp finely chopped coriander, plus extra leaves to serve

1cm piece of ginger, finely grated

2 garlic cloves, finely grated

1 red chilli, deseeded and finely chopped, plus 1 extra chilli, sliced, to serve

12 lettuce leaves (I like butter lettuce or baby gem)

salt and black pepper

Put the chicken breasts into a sauté pan and just cover with cold water. Add the soy sauce and place over a low heat. Bring to simmering point then gently poach for 15 minutes until cooked through, adding the green beans for the last 3 minutes of cooking.

While the chicken is cooking, heat the butter and olive oil in a frying pan over a medium heat and add the onion. Cook for about 10 minutes until golden.

Remove the sauté pan from the heat and use a slotted spoon to remove the green beans. Plunge them into a bowl of really cold water – this prevents them from going soggy and keeps them nice and green. Once cold, dry the beans on some kitchen paper and keep to one side.

Allow the chicken to cool in the poaching liquid for around 15 minutes, then remove it to a chopping board. Use two forks to shred it, then allow to cool to room temperature.

Put the lime juice, yoghurt and hoisin sauce in a large mixing bowl. Add the spring onions, coriander, ginger, garlic and chopped chilli, and mix well.

Add the shredded chicken and beans to the bowl, along with some seasoning, and toss everything together lightly to combine.

Divide the mixture evenly between the lettuce leaves and top with a few extra coriander leaves and some chilli slices.

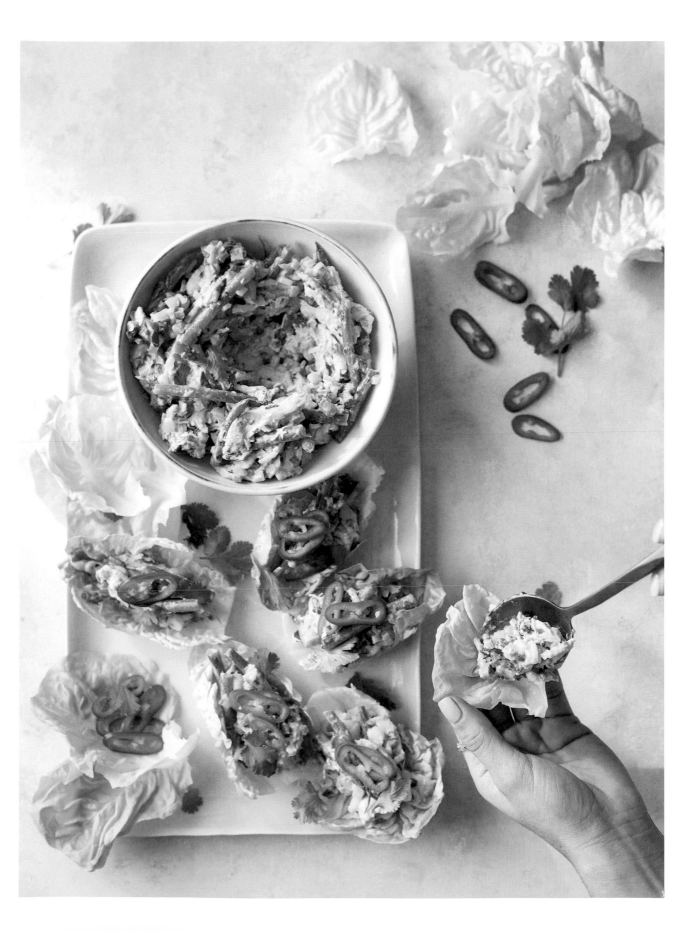

# coriander lime prawns with pineapple, pea & chilli rice

This Asian-inspired dish combines lots of incredible flavours. I have always admired this style of cooking because it's very simple. Something about pineapple and prawns just works. I added chilli rice to this dish because it's important to include a carbohydrate element to give you energy and fill you up.

**serves 2**

200g raw prawns, deveined
1 tbsp roughly chopped coriander
finely grated zest and juice of 1 lime
1 tbsp olive oil
80g easy-cook brown rice
1 red onion, finely chopped
100g fresh pineapple, cut into chunks
70g peas (fresh or frozen)
1 red chilli, deseeded and finely
  chopped
salt and black pepper

**to serve**
lime wedges
coriander leaves

> **< TIP >**
> **The lime cuts through the sweetness of the pineapple so don't hold back!**

Place the raw prawns in a mixing bowl and add the coriander, lime zest, juice and half the olive oil. Mix well and pop into the fridge to marinate while you make the rice.

Place the rice in a saucepan and rinse under cold water, then drain and cover with fresh water. Bring to the boil over a medium–high heat then pop a lid on, reduce the heat to a simmer and cook for around 20–25 minutes, or until done (check the packet instructions).

Once the rice is cooked, drain into a sieve or colander and keep handy. Rinse the saucepan then return it to the heat. Add the remaining oil and the red onion. Gently fry the onion for 4–5 minutes until it has started to soften, then add the pineapple, peas and chilli. Reduce the heat and cook for another 3 minutes.

Return the rice to the pan and mix well. Turn the heat right down to keep everything hot, but not cooking, while you cook the prawns.

Heat a frying pan over a high heat then add the prawns, tipping any marinade left in the bowl into the pan. Cook for around 5 minutes, turning occasionally, until they have gone pink, curled up and are cooked through.

Divide the rice between two bowls and top with the prawns. Serve with a good squeeze of lime and some coriander leaves.

# goat's cheese, spinach & asparagus frittata

I am a huge fan of eggs so having a lunch recipe dedicated to them was inevitable. My frittata is a sort of glorified omelette with a combination of light and fluffy eggs and creamy goat's cheese – I like to serve it straight out of the pan.

## makes 8 wedges

4 new potatoes, sliced into 5mm rounds
1 tbsp olive oil
1 red onion, chopped
8 asparagus tips
80g spinach leaves
6 large eggs
40g goat's cheese
salt and black pepper

Preheat your oven to 200°C/180°C fan/gas 6.

Put the potato slices in a saucepan and cover with cold water. Bring to the boil on a medium–high heat then reduce the heat and simmer for 5–6 minutes, until the potatoes are just tender all the way through when pierced with a sharp knife. Drain and keep to one side.

Heat an ovenproof frying pan on a medium heat and add the olive oil. Add the red onion and fry for 3 minutes until it has started to soften. Add the asparagus tips and cook for a further 3 minutes. Add the spinach leaves and cook until they have just wilted – this will only take a minute. Then add the potato slices. Mix everything together and season well.

Crack the eggs into a large jug and beat with a fork.

Tip the beaten egg into the pan to cover the veg, gently stirring and lifting the veg to make sure the egg gets all around and down to the bottom of the pan. Distribute the vegetables evenly then break the goat's cheese into pieces and drop into the egg mix. Use the back of a spoon to press the cheese into the egg if you need to.

Transfer the frying pan to the oven for 12–15 minutes, until the frittata is golden brown, with no runny egg left. Remove from the oven and allow to cool in the pan for 5 minutes before sliding it out onto a chopping board.

This is great with a green salad or some steamed greens if you want to make it a little more substantial.

# courgette, walnut & ricotta quiche with a quinoa crust

I first tried a quinoa-based quiche in a café in Chelsea and I wasn't sure if it was something that would easily translate to my own cooking skills. I was amazed the first time I tried to cook it – and it had an even bake! This makes eight portions, so either share it or keep it to eat over a few days.

## serves 8

### for the crust

1 tsp olive oil
300g cooked quinoa (about 100g uncooked)
1 egg, lightly beaten
2 tsp mustard powder
2 tbsp finely chopped parsley
salt and black pepper

### for the filling

1 tbsp olive oil
1 onion, diced
3 garlic cloves, finely grated
2 courgettes, grated
10g sprigs of thyme, leaves picked
180g ricotta
½ tsp freshly grated nutmeg
4 large eggs, beaten
40g walnuts, roughly chopped
20g Parmesan, finely grated

Preheat your oven to 180°C/160°C fan/gas 4. Lightly grease a 23cm quiche/tart/pie tin with the olive oil and keep handy. Place the cooked quinoa in a mixing bowl and add the beaten egg, mustard powder, parsley and some seasoning. Mix everything together well and then tip it all into the prepared tin. Use the back of a spoon to spread it out to line the tin, being sure to leave no holes, and to take it up the sides. Press it down firmly to pack it together and make your quiche crust.

Bake it in the oven for 15–18 minutes until it is golden brown and the base feels dried out to the touch. Leave to one side to cool while you assemble the filling.

Heat the olive oil in a frying pan and add the onion. Cook, stirring often, for 5 minutes until it is softened and starting to turn golden. Add the garlic and stir for another 30 seconds.

Give the grated courgette a good squeeze to remove some of the excess water and then add to the pan along with the thyme leaves. Cook for another 5 minutes then remove from the heat and transfer to a large mixing bowl to cool.

Add the ricotta to the courgette and onion mix once it has cooled, and stir well. Add the nutmeg, eggs and some salt and pepper, and stir well to combine, then pour the mixture into your quinoa crust. Sprinkle the walnuts and Parmesan over the top and pop it into the oven to bake for around 25 minutes.

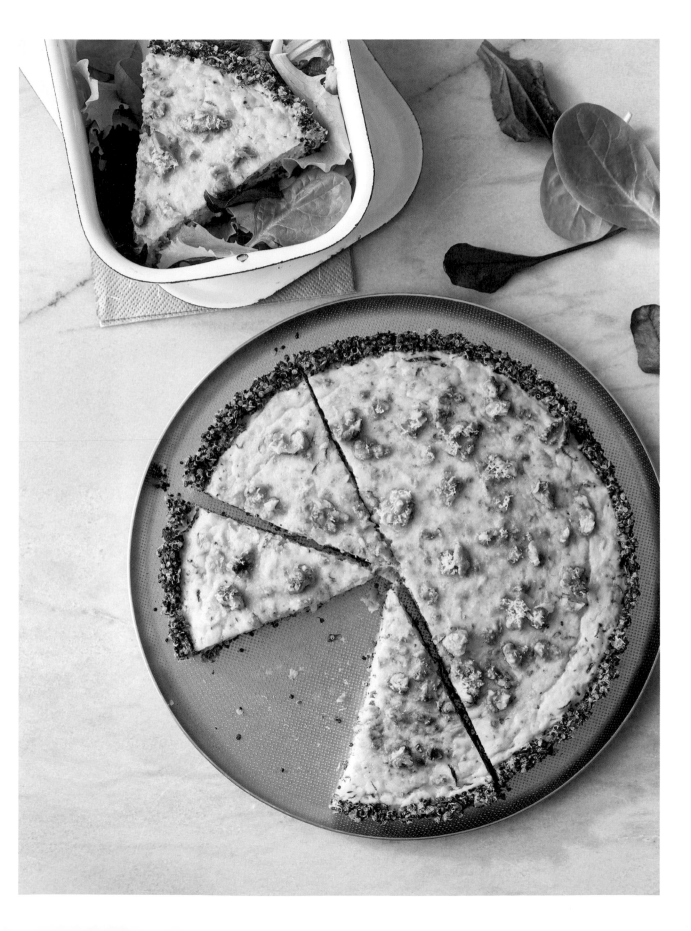

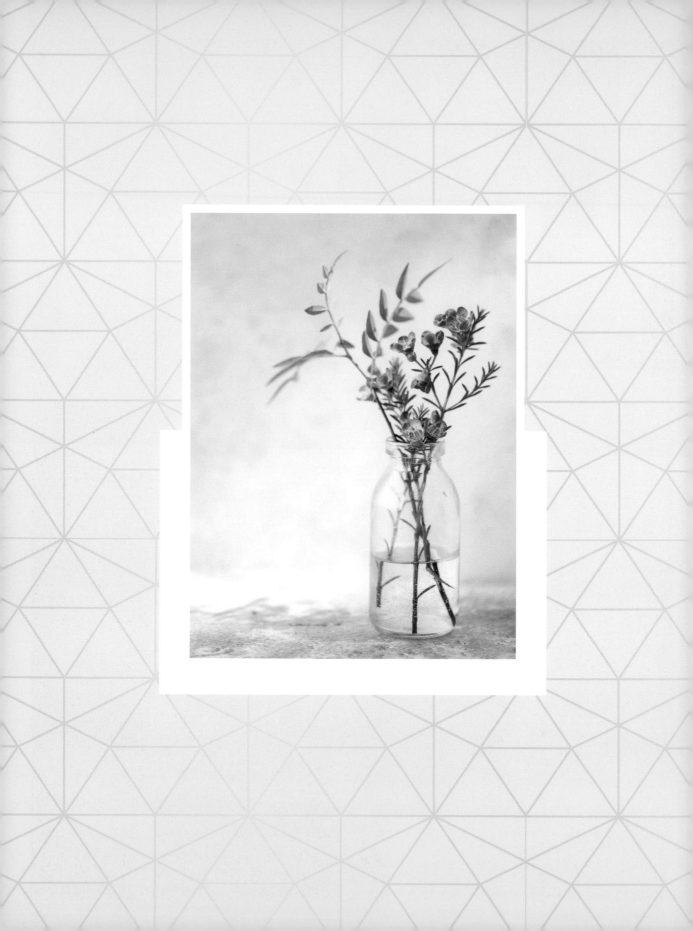

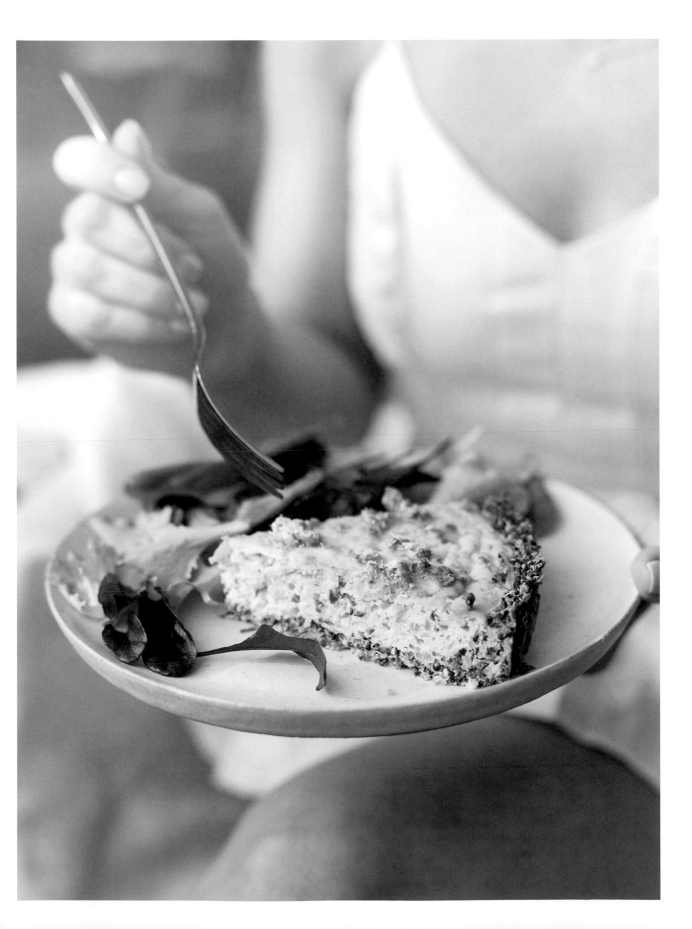

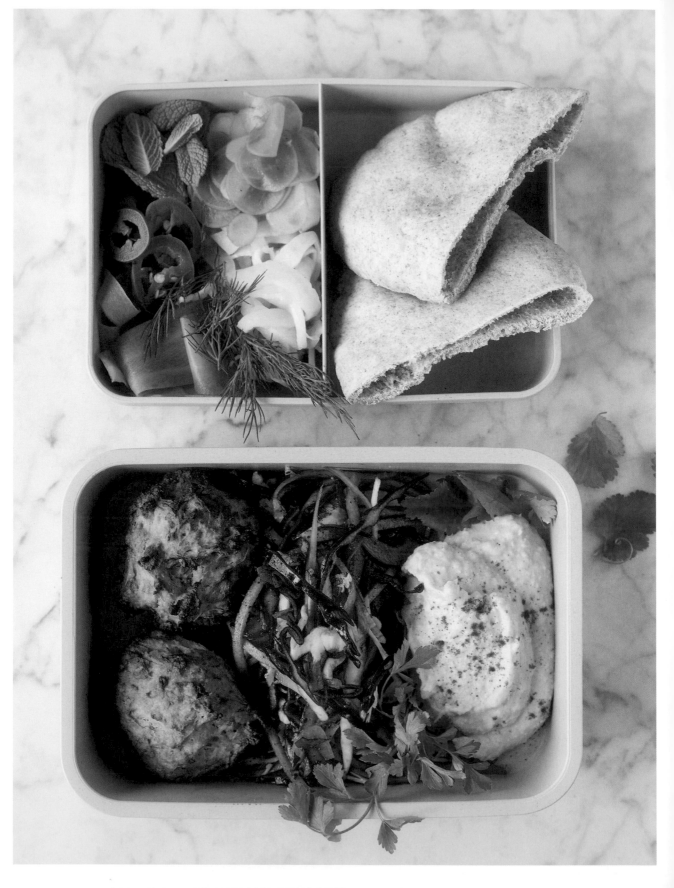

# mediterranean lunchbox

**pack up & go** OPTION

This flavour combo is the dream. They are all fairly simple to make but create impact when served together. If you're not packing it into a lunchbox, serve everything on a lovely big sharing platter, with the falafel, hummus, slaw, quick pickles, warm flatbreads and a whole load of fresh herbs.

**serves 6**

## sweet potato falafel

1 tbsp olive oil

about 400g sweet potato (1 large or 2 small)

2 garlic cloves, crushed to a paste

1 tsp ground cumin

2 tbsp finely chopped coriander

juice of ½ lemon

150g chickpea flour

salt and black pepper

**to serve**

wholemeal pitta breads or flatbreads

herbs, such as mint, coriander, parsley and dill

Preheat the oven to 200°C/180°C fan/gas 6 and line a baking sheet with non-stick baking paper. Use the oil to lightly grease the paper to make sure nothing sticks.

Either microwave the sweet potato for 4 minutes on each side (I like microwaving it because it is by far the quickest way to soften it if you're impatient) or bake in the hot oven for 40 minutes (or until a skewer goes through easily).

Once it is cool enough to handle, peel off the skin, discard and place the potato in a mixing bowl. Add the garlic, cumin, coriander, lemon juice and chickpea flour. Season with a little salt and pepper then mash everything together into a thick paste.

Use a tablespoon to scoop up equal-sized pieces, and use your hands to shape them into rough balls, placing them on the baking sheet as you go. If the mixture is sticking to you, dampen your hands with a little water.

Bake the falafel in the oven for 15 minutes, then flip them over and cook the other side for 10–15 minutes. You want them to be golden brown and crisp all over.

## hummus

1 x 400g tin chickpeas, drained
and rinsed
2 tbsp tahini
4 roasted garlic cloves (put raw
cloves in their skins on the tray with
the falafel for 20 minutes)
juice of 1 lemon
3 tbsp extra virgin olive oil, plus extra
to serve
1 tsp ground cumin
a pinch of cayenne pepper
a pinch of paprika, plus extra to
serve
a pinch of salt

Put the chickpeas into the large bowl of a food processor. If you have more time and want to make the ultimate hummus, then pop the chickpeas out of their skins before adding to the food processor.

Add the tahini, roasted garlic cloves (popped out of their skins), lemon juice, extra virgin olive oil, cumin, cayenne, paprika and salt. Blitz everything for 1 minute then pause, scrape the sides down and blend again until it is silky smooth.

Taste the hummus and adjust the seasoning if you need to. Give it one last blitz and then transfer to a serving dish. Use a spoon to swirl a pattern in the top and drizzle over a little more extra virgin olive oil and a pinch of paprika.

## rainbow slaw

½ small red cabbage, shredded
½ small white cabbage, shredded
2 carrots, julienned
1 red pepper, halved, deseeded and
very finely sliced
1 red onion, very finely sliced
juice of 2 lemons
3 tbsp extra virgin olive oil
1 tbsp chopped coriander
1 tbsp chopped parsley
1 tbsp sumac
a pinch of salt

Place all the vegetables in a large mixing bowl and use your hands to lift and mix it all together. Squeeze over the lemon juice, drizzle over the olive oil, add the herbs, sumac and salt. Stir everything together until it is all coated in the dressing.

## quick pickles

3 tbsp red wine vinegar
1 tbsp salt
1 tbsp coriander seeds
boiling water, to cover

You can quick-pickle anything you like in around 15 minutes. It will keep in the fridge for up to 5 days, but will get softer. Use the above volumes in clean, airtight containers on each of the following (or a combination of whatever you fancy):

2 carrots, peeled into ribbons
2 red onions, very thinly sliced
200g radishes, thinly sliced
1 fennel bulb, very thinly sliced
4 jalapeños (or other chillies), thinly sliced

# spiced courgette, spinach & coconut soup

Coconut milk is the base for many of my homemade soups because it is rich and creamy. I also adore the colour of this pretty green soup.

**serves 4**

2 tsp olive oil
1 onion, finely chopped
3 garlic cloves, finely grated
1 tsp ground cumin
1 tsp ground coriander
1 tsp chipotle chilli flakes
4 courgettes, grated
250g spinach leaves
1 x 400ml tin reduced-fat
   coconut milk
250ml vegetable stock
salt and black pepper

Heat the olive oil in a large saucepan and add the onion. Cook for 10 minutes over a low heat to bring out the natural sweetness. Add the garlic, cumin, coriander and chilli flakes and cook for a further 2 minutes, stirring frequently so nothing sticks or burns.

Add the grated courgette and mix well to make sure it gets coated in the spices. Cook for 8–10 minutes so some of the water from the courgette evaporates and the flavour intensifies. Once the courgette has softened right down and become a golden brown, add the spinach leaves. Stir until they have wilted then add the coconut milk and stock.

Allow everything to simmer together for 5–6 minutes.

Season with salt and pepper (you may not need any salt as the stock will make it quite salty already) and use a stick blender to make a lovely smooth, tasty soup with a bit of a chilli kick.

**< TIP >**
**This also makes a really nice starter if you're having a dinner party.**

# pack-up-and-go chicken pho

Anyone that knows me knows how obsessed I am with Vietnamese food. It's amazing how much flavour you can pack into a clear broth while keeping it super healthy. Of course, you can make this in a bowl if you don't want to take it with you, but I love how practical it is to travel with. Feel free to mix up the vegetables. I also like to replace the chicken with prawns to keep a good balance between meat and seafood throughout the week.

**serves 1**

2 tsp bouillon powder
1cm piece of ginger, finely chopped
1 tbsp low-salt soy sauce
2 tsp fish sauce
finely grated zest and juice of 1 lime
1 red Thai chilli, finely chopped
60g wide brown rice noodles
1 carrot, spiralised
20g sugar snaps, sliced
150g cooked chicken breast, shredded
1 spring onion, thinly sliced
1 tbsp mint leaves
1 tbsp coriander leaves
450ml boiling water

Put the bouillon powder, ginger, soy sauce, fish sauce, lime zest and juice into a 1-litre jar or airtight container.

Add the chilli, rice noodles, carrot, sugar snaps and cooked chicken breast. If you're taking this to the office, pop the spring onion and herbs in a little bag and pop that on top of the chicken to add later, so they stay fresh.

When you are ready to eat, add the boiling water to the container. Allow everything to sit for 10–12 minutes so the noodles cook in the boiling water. Then gently stir with your chopsticks to mix around into a delicious broth.

Add the spring onion and herbs. Add more lime if you like a sour kick alongside the heat.

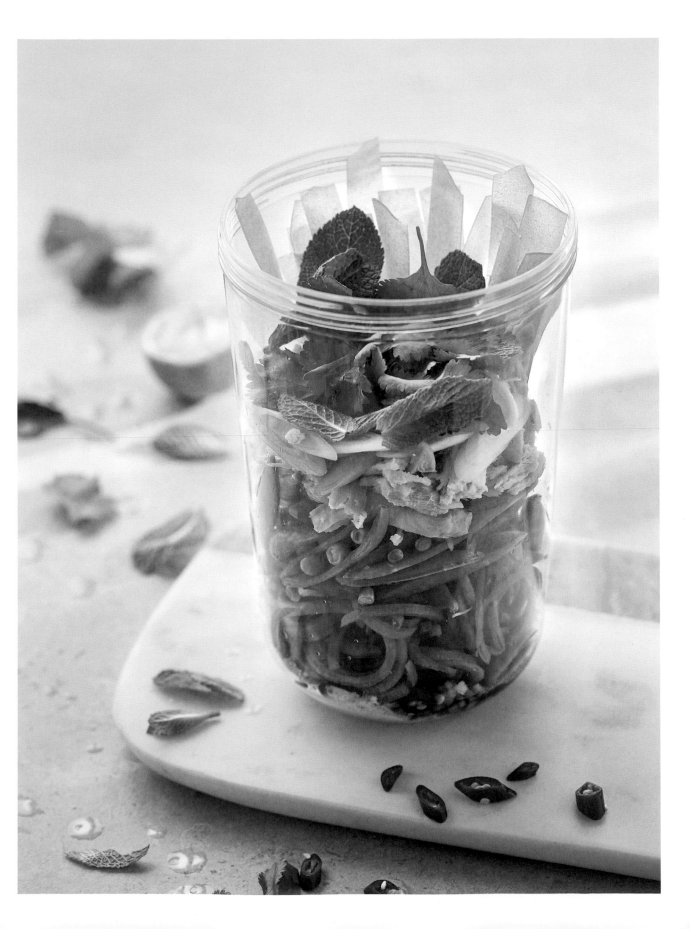

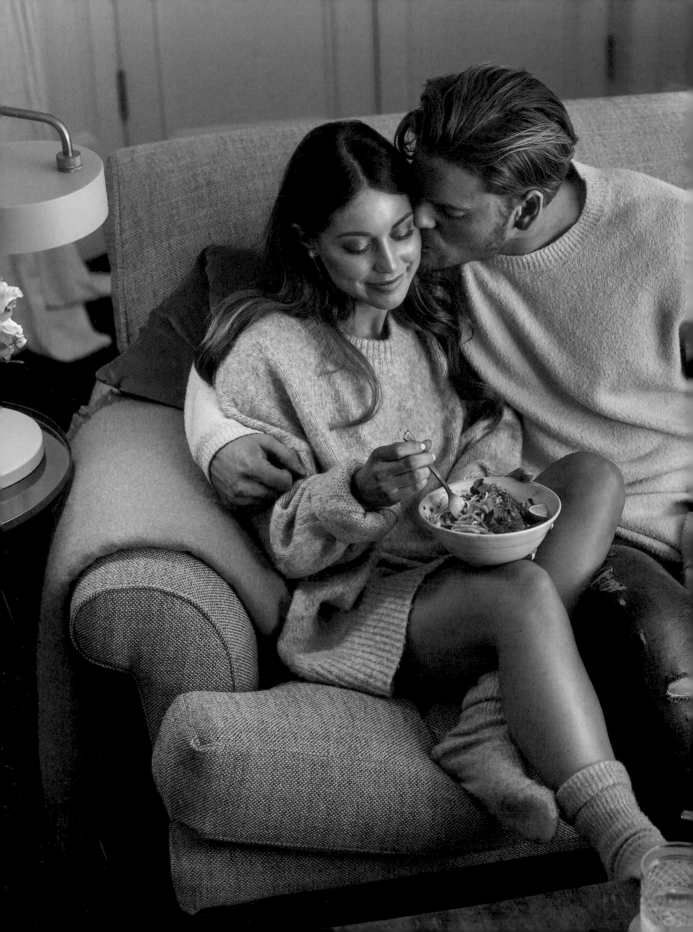

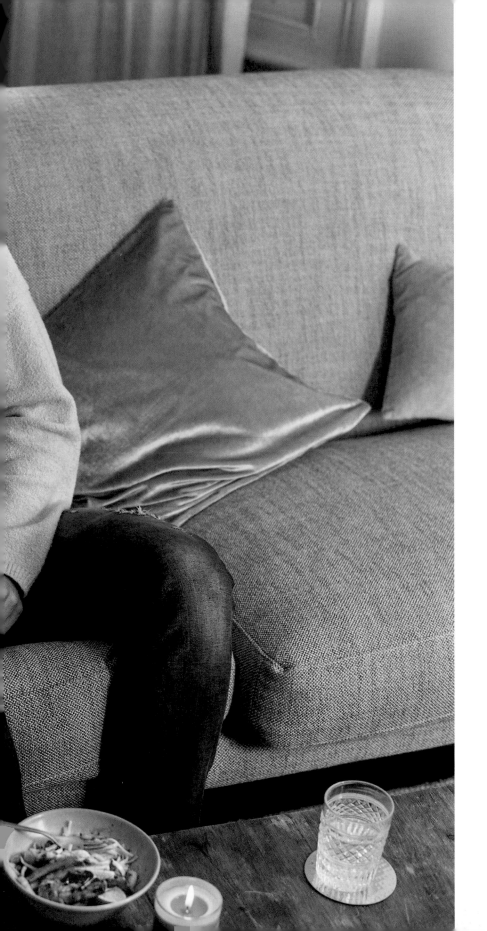

dinner

# one-tray roast chicken

If I'm having people round for a Sunday roast, I will often cook this with the dauphinoise potatoes on the next page, but it's a perfect supper on its own too (with minimal washing up). If you are cooking the two dishes together, I suggest you make the dauphinoise first and prep the chicken and veg whilst it's baking. The dauphinoise will hold together really well and then you can just give them a final blast in the oven under the veg tray for 10 minutes to heat up again while the chicken rests.

## serves 6-8

1 large free-range chicken (about 1.8kg)

2 bay leaves

10g sprigs of thyme

2 tbsp wholegrain mustard

1 tbsp runny honey

750g sweet potatoes, cut into wedges (optional – if you're serving with the dauphinoise you won't need these as well)

350g baby parsnips, cut into halves or quarters, depending on size

350g baby carrots, halved lengthways

2 tbsp olive oil (optional)

salt and black pepper

Preheat the oven to 190°C/170°C fan/gas 5 and line a large roasting tin with non-stick baking paper.

Place the chicken in the tin and stuff the bay leaves and thyme into the cavity. Put the mustard and honey on top of the breasts and use your hands to rub them all over, making sure not to miss the wings or legs. Add a little seasoning and roast in the oven for 45 minutes.

Remove from the oven and spoon the mustard and honey dressing over the chicken to baste it. Add the prepared root veg to the tin all around the chicken and turn them over in all the cooking juices to coat it. If you need a little more to coat everything, then use the olive oil.

Return the tin to the oven for another 15 minutes, then remove and turn the veg. Place back in the oven for another 15 minutes.

By this point the chicken should be beautifully golden and cooked through. To check it is cooked, poke a skewer or a knife into the thickest part and if the juices run clear, it is ready. Remove from the oven, lift the chicken out and place on a large plate to rest. Turn the oven up to 220°C/200°C fan/gas 7.

Slide the veg off the baking paper back into the tin, give everything a final shake and return to the oven for a final 10 minutes.

Remove the veg from the oven and either return the chicken to carve in the tin or decant the veg as well and serve everything up on a large platter.

This is also lovely with some simply steamed greens like Tenderstem broccoli, green beans, asparagus or sugar snaps.

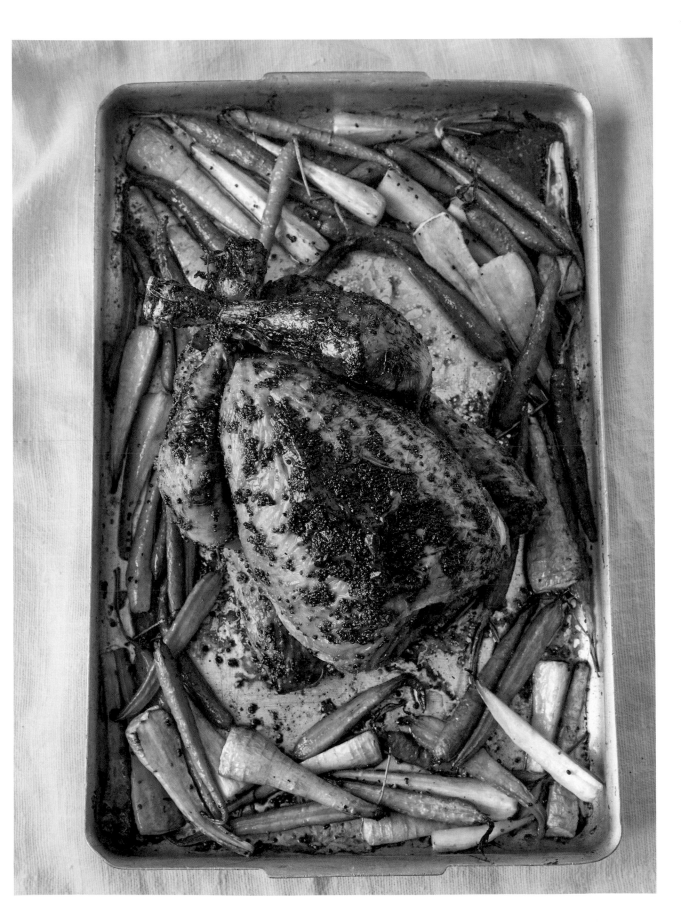

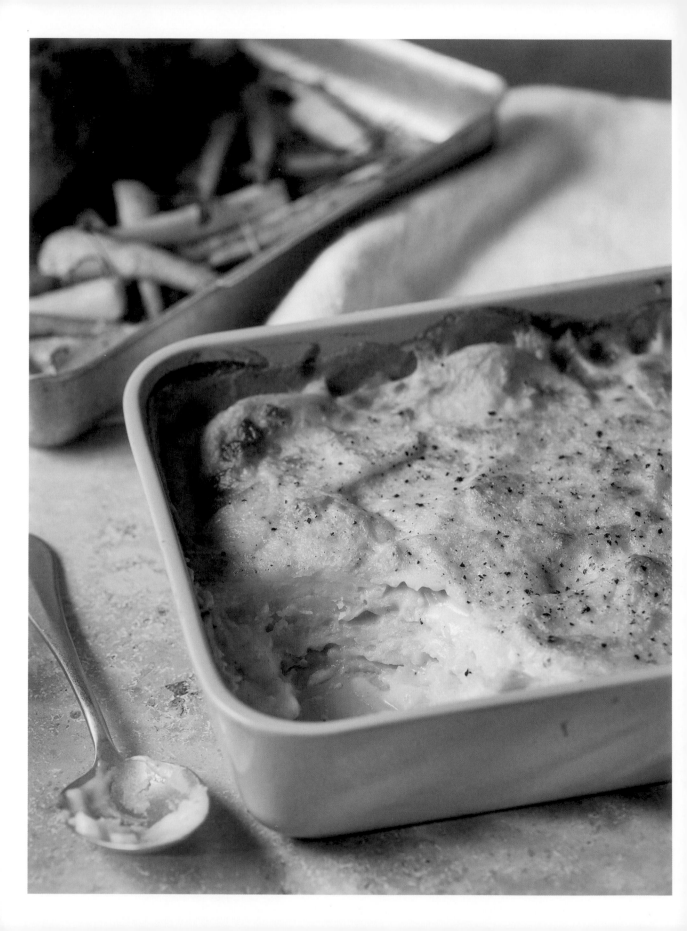

# lower-fat dauphinoise potatoes

This dish is deceptively easy despite being served at the most sophisticated of dinner parties. Because I love them so much I created this *slightly* healthier option for you guys. One of the things that is useful about these potatoes is that they keep really well in the fridge so you can tuck in the next day too – although chances are there won't be any leftovers.

## serves 6-8

50g butter

45g brown rice flour

350ml whole milk

350ml skimmed milk

3 garlic cloves, bashed

¼ tsp freshly grated nutmeg

1kg potatoes, peeled and thinly sliced (ideally on a mandoline)

40g Gruyère, grated (optional)

salt and black pepper

Preheat your oven to 180°C/160°C fan/gas 4 and use 5g of the butter to lightly grease a baking dish, approximately 18 x 28cm.

Put the remaining butter in a saucepan and add the brown rice flour, both milks and the bashed garlic cloves (you'll remove these later). Place over a medium–low heat and start to whisk everything together. You need to keep gently whisking all the time. The butter will melt and after about 5 minutes or so it will start to thicken. Cook for another 2 minutes and then take off the heat, whisk in the nutmeg and season to taste. Keep to one side.

Bring a large saucepan of water to the boil with a pinch of salt added. Once it is boiling, carefully slide in the potato slices and cook for 3 minutes. Drain and allow them to steam dry for a minute or two before returning them to their saucepan. Remove the garlic cloves from the sauce and pour the sauce all over the potatoes, gently stirring them so they are all coated.

Transfer the potatoes to the buttered baking dish, levelling them out as you go. Pour over any remaining sauce in the pan and give the dish a little wobble to help it all level out.

Sprinkle over the grated cheese, if using, and pop the dish into the oven for 30 minutes until golden. Remove from the oven and use a skewer to check that the potatoes are cooked through. If not, return to the oven for another 10 minutes.

Take out of the oven and rest for 10 minutes before serving.

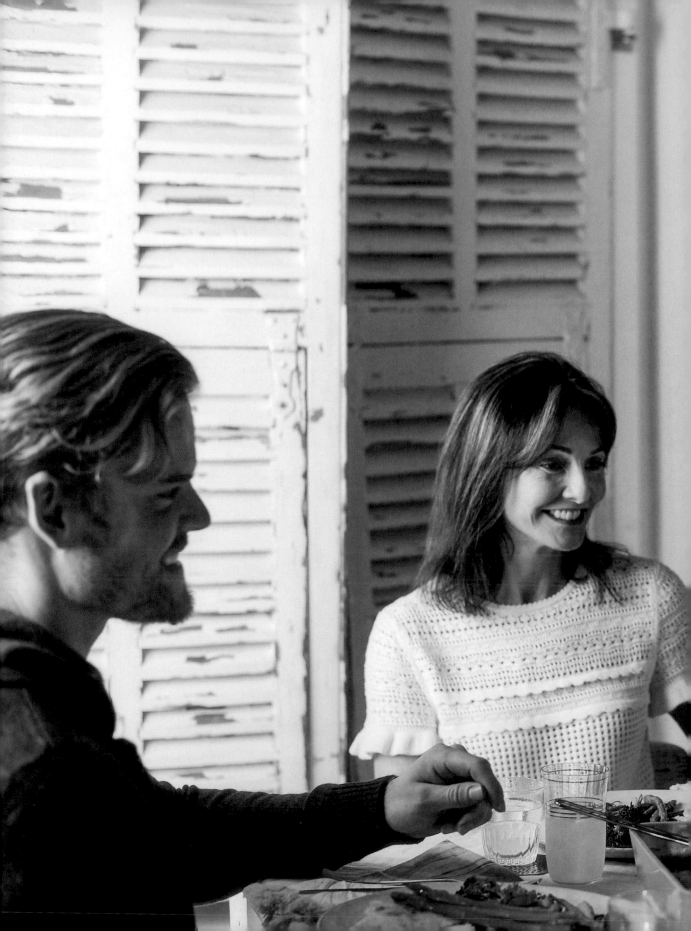

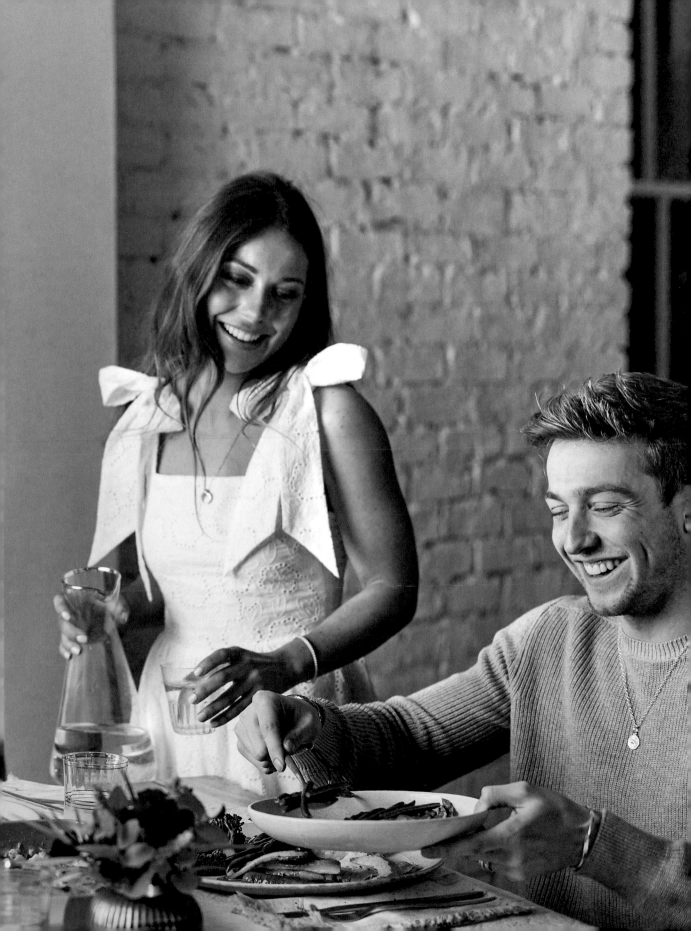

# turkey kofte with yoghurt dipping sauce & red onion & feta salad

Turkey is a brilliant low-fat lean meat choice that tends to be overlooked except on Christmas Day. I think people are put off from integrating it into their daily diet because Christmas Day turkey often ends up dry due to stressed cooking conditions. This recipe will bring turkey back to the forefront of your kitchen because it is truly mouth-watering.

## serves 2

### for the kofte
300g turkey thigh mince
½ red onion, finely chopped
2 garlic cloves, finely grated
1 tbsp roughly chopped coriander
1 tbsp roughly chopped parsley
1 tbsp harissa paste
salt and black pepper

### for the dipping sauce
2 tbsp Greek yoghurt
juice of 1 lemon
1 tbsp finely chopped dill

### for the salad
60g mixed salad leaves
½ red onion, finely sliced
20g feta, crumbled
a few parsley leaves

Preheat your oven to 210°C/190°C fan/gas 6½ and line a baking sheet with non-stick baking paper.

Place all the ingredients for the kofte in a large mixing bowl, with a good pinch each of salt and pepper, and use your hands to squeeze and mix everything together. You want everything to be really well mixed. Divide the mixture into 4 and shape into long sausage shapes, placing them on the lined baking sheet as you go. Pop them into the oven and bake for 25 minutes, until golden brown.

While the kofte are baking, make the dipping sauce by mixing everything together in a small dish, with salt and pepper to taste.

Put the salad leaves onto your serving plate then scatter over the chopped onion and crumbled feta, layering up as you go. Add the parsley leaves for a final flourish.

Serve the salad alongside the turkey kofte and yoghurt dipping sauce.

# vegetable thai curry

I'm trying to include more vegetable-based meals in my diet. If I use interesting vegetables with good texture, such as baby corn, I find I get the same amount of satisfaction as I do from eating meat and I don't even notice it is missing. For me this recipe is all about the sauce and I guarantee a homemade curry sauce has tonnes more flavour than a takeaway version.

## serves 2

2 tsp olive oil
1 small aubergine, cut into chunks
6 baby corn, cut into chunks
100g green beans, cut into 3cm
  lengths
1 courgette, cut into chunks
400ml reduced-fat coconut milk

### for the curry paste

1 banana shallot, roughly chopped
2 kaffir lime leaves, torn into pieces
1 red chilli, roughly chopped
1 lemongrass stalk, outer layers
  removed then roughly chopped
2cm piece of ginger, peeled and
  roughly chopped
2 garlic cloves, roughly chopped
2 tbsp roughly chopped coriander
  leaves
1 tbsp low-salt soy sauce
50ml water

### to serve

a handful of Thai basil leaves
lime wedges

Start by placing all the ingredients for the curry paste in a food processor and blitzing to a paste, stopping to scrape the sides down a couple of times to make sure everything is included.

Heat the olive oil in a large saucepan or wok. Add the curry paste and cook for 2 minutes until it is very aromatic, then add the aubergine and corn and cook for another 3 minutes. Add the green beans, courgette and coconut milk then reduce the heat and simmer for around 15 minutes, stirring occasionally.

Divide the curry between two bowls and top with a few Thai basil leaves. A squeeze of fresh lime is also a nice addition.

# warm barley salad with pomegranate & feta

Barley has a unique flavour with a moreish chewy texture. The combination of ingredients here make this a sensational looking Instagram-worthy salad and the pomegranate jewels add a gourmet crunch.

## serves 2

100g pearl barley
600ml vegetable stock or water
60g pomegranate seeds
3 spring onions, thinly sliced
40g watercress
40g baby leaves, to include spinach and rocket
40g feta
30g pistachios, chopped

### for the dressing
2 tbsp finely chopped dill
2 tbsp finely chopped parsley
juice of 1 lemon
1 tbsp pomegranate molasses
1 ½ tbsp extra-virgin olive oil
salt and black pepper

Rinse the pearl barley under cold running water and put it into a saucepan. Add the stock or water and bring up to simmering point over a medium heat. Once it is simmering, cook for 50 minutes, or until al dente, then drain in a colander and leave to steam dry.

Place all the dressing ingredients in a small bowl and whisk together.

Put the pearl barley into a mixing bowl and pour the dressing over the grains. Give everything a good stir to coat all the barley.

Add the pomegranate seeds and spring onions and mix lightly.

Divide the watercress and salad leaves between two plates and top with the pearl barley mix. Crumble over the feta and top with some chopped pistachios.

< TIP >
**This isn't a salad for tossing because you will lose all the exciting ingredients to the bottom.**

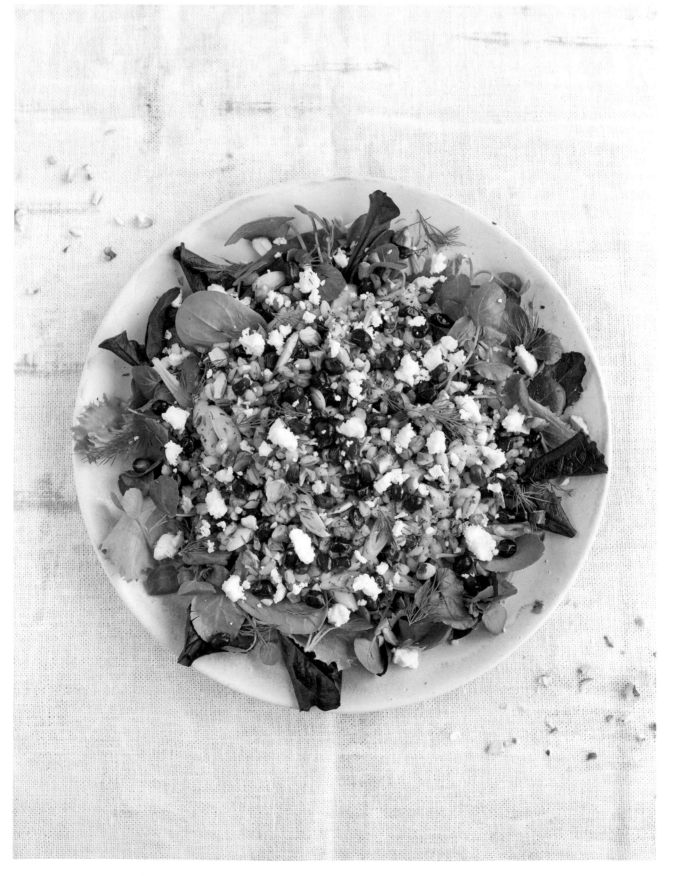

# tofu stir-fry

If I could I would eat rice noodles every day. In my early days of cooking I would experiment with stir-fries at my mum's house and the core ingredient was always rice noodles. Then I would add a dash of this and a dash of that and it always turned out pretty well! Since then I've learnt I used to use WAY too many salty ingredients in one dish so here is a lighter version. When tofu is cooked well it is a delicious way to add protein to a meal. I like to fry the tofu until it is really golden and crispy. If it doesn't work for you, substitute the tofu for chicken.

## serves 2

15g cashew nuts

2 tsp sesame seeds

100g flat rice noodles

1½ tbsp toasted sesame oil

6 Tenderstem broccoli stems

1 red pepper, deseeded and cut into strips

1 carrot, peeled into thin ribbons

40g kale, leaves torn and tough stalks removed

4 spring onions, finely sliced

2 garlic cloves, thinly sliced

1 tbsp low-salt soy sauce

2 tbsp sriracha

1 tbsp runny honey

150g firm tofu, cubed

1 tbsp cornflour

1 lime, cut into wedges, to serve

Toast the cashews in a dry frying pan on a low heat for 4–5 minutes, tossing frequently so they don't burn. Remove to a chopping board then add the sesame seeds to the pan. Toast in the same way – they will take a little less time so keep your eye on them. Tip onto a plate. Roughly chop the cashews and set both aside.

Bring a large pan of water to the boil, add the noodles and cook for 4 minutes (or according to the packet instructions) until they are al dente. Drain, rinse thoroughly under cold water and keep to one side.

Heat about half of the sesame oil in a wok or large frying pan over a high heat. Add the broccoli, red pepper, carrot, kale, spring onions and garlic. Cook over a high heat, tossing the pan, for 5 minutes. Add the drained noodles to the vegetables then add the soy sauce, sriracha and honey and toss for 1 minute to coat the noodles. Remove from the heat and keep to one side while you cook the tofu.

Place the tofu cubes in a bowl, add the cornflour and toss the cubes until they are well coated in the cornflour. Heat the remaining sesame oil in a separate frying pan. Add the tofu and cook until pale golden and crisp, tossing the plan to turn the cubes frequently and cook on all sides. Add the tofu to the stir-fry along with the cashew nuts and sesame seeds.

Divide between two serving plates and serve immediately, with a couple of lime wedges.

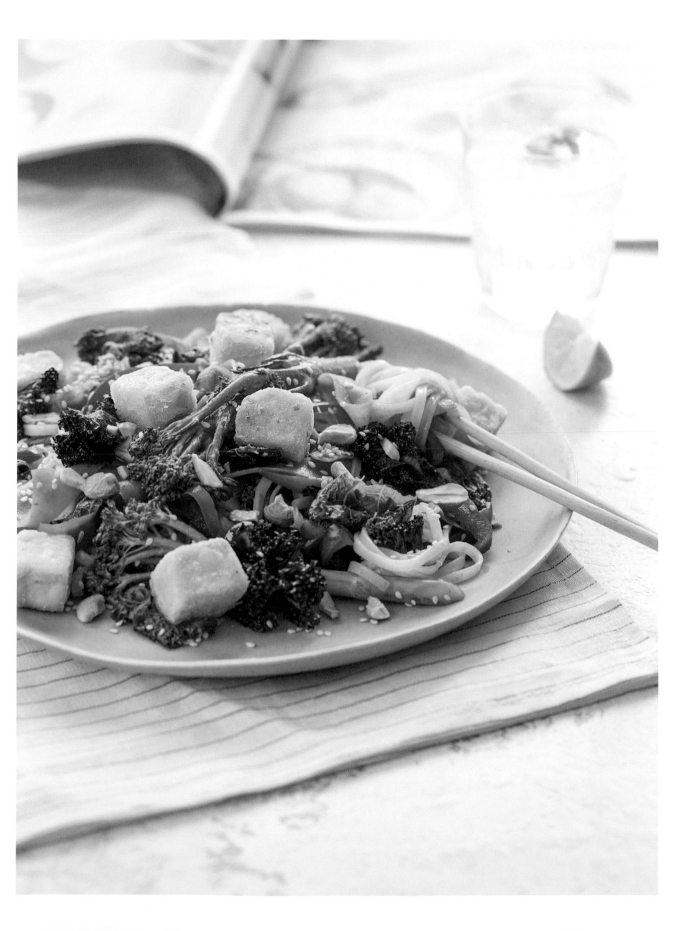

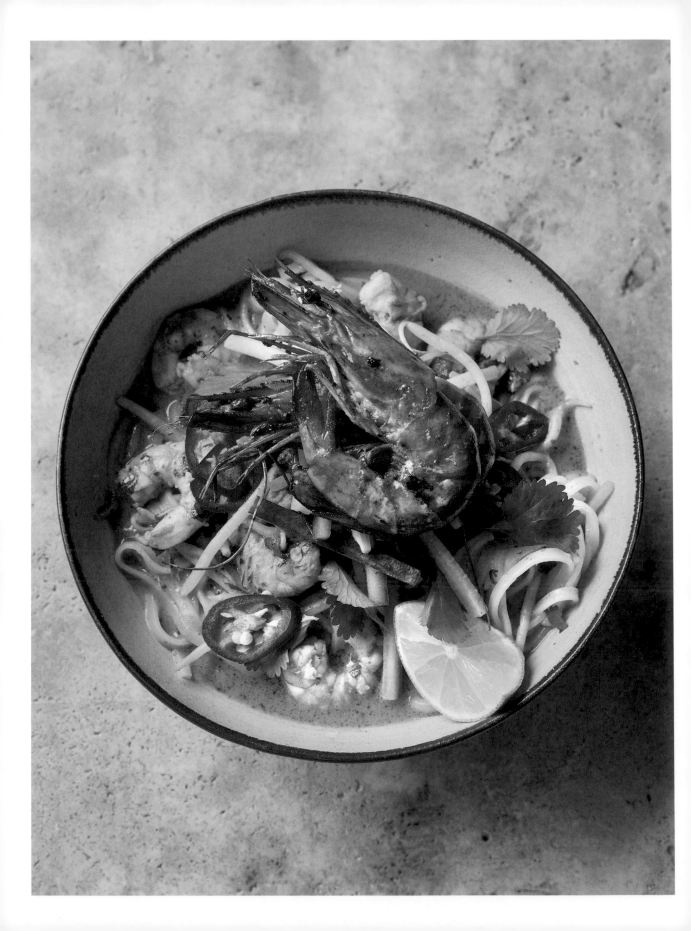

# spicy prawn laksa

This is one of Ryan's FAVOURITES so it's a regular on our table at home, he isn't the greatest with hot food, so I don't go mad on the chillies! The soupy element to this dish makes it super filling and to save money I buy frozen prawns and keep them in the freezer for when I need them.

## serves 2

2 tsp olive oil

1 tbsp red Thai curry paste

3 tbsp laksa paste (or use an extra 3 tbsp red Thai curry paste if you can't get it)

1 x 400ml tin reduced-fat coconut milk

2 tsp fish sauce

300ml vegetable stock

120g medium rice noodles

200g raw, shelled king prawns, deveined, plus 4 raw shell-on king prawns

80g beansprouts

2 tbsp coriander leaves

2 red chillies, thinly sliced (deseeded for less heat if you prefer)

¼ cucumber, cut into 4mm batons

1 lime, cut into wedges

Heat 1 teaspoon of the oil in a wok and add the Thai curry and laksa pastes. Cook for 2 minutes until aromatic. Slowly add the coconut milk to the paste, stirring it in with each addition until it is fully mixed in, then add the fish sauce and stock and let everything simmer for 10 minutes.

Boil a kettle and put the rice noodles into a heatproof bowl or saucepan. Once the water has boiled, cover the noodles and soak for around 7 minutes (or according to the packet instructions). Once they have softened, drain and rinse under cold water and keep to one side.

Add the shelled prawns and beansprouts to the wok. Roughly chop three quarters of the coriander leaves and add those to the wok as well. Reduce the heat to as low as it will go and let the prawns and beansprouts cook for 4–5 minutes.

In the meantime, toss the shell-on prawns in the remaining teaspoon of oil and heat a griddle or frying pan over a high heat. Add the prawns and cook for 3 minutes each side, or until cooked through.

Stir the chillies into the laksa, reserving a few slices to garnish.

Add the noodles to the sauce and stir gently. Remove from the heat.

Divide the laksa between two bowls and top with the cucumber batons. Add 2 shell-on prawns to each bowl, the reserved chilli slices and the remaining coriander leaves. Serve with plenty of lime wedges.

# lasagne with loads of veggies

The ultimate comfort food. As part of my ongoing resolution in life to eat more vegetables, I created this flavoursome vegetable-packed lasagne recipe. In order to concoct the best lasagne recipe ever it is crucial to perfect the Bolognese sauce using a combo of oregano, basil, tomato and garlic for flavour.

## serves 6

2 tbsp olive oil

1 butternut squash, peeled, deseeded and cut into long, thin slices around 1mm thick

1 red onion, diced

2 celery sticks, diced

1 large carrot, peeled and diced

1 aubergine, peeled and diced

500g beef mince (5% fat)

1 tbsp tomato purée

3 garlic cloves, finely grated

1 tbsp dried oregano

1 tsp freshly ground nutmeg

2 x 400g tins chopped tomatoes

2 tbsp roughly chopped basil

45g butter

45g brown rice flour

600ml skimmed milk

salt and black pepper

Preheat your oven to 220°C/200°C fan/gas 7 and line two roasting tins with non-stick baking paper. Have ready a lasagne or baking dish, about 28 x 18cm (or a round one with a similar capacity). Brush the butternut squash slices with 1 tablespoon of the oil, placing them in a single layer in one of the roasting tins as you go (you'll need to do two batches, so set aside those that don't fit).

Put the diced onion, celery, carrot and aubergine in the other roasting tin and drizzle over ½ tablespoon of the oil. Place both tins in the hot oven and roast for 10 minutes, then remove the tins, turn the diced veg and return that tin to the oven. Remove the squash from the tin and add the rest of the slices to the tin. Roast for 10–15 minutes until all the veg are tender. Remove from the oven and reduce the oven temperature to 180°C/160°C fan/gas 4.

Heat the remaining ½ tablespoon of oil in a large saucepan and cook the beef mince, stirring, for 5 minutes until browned all over. Stir in the tomato purée and garlic and cook for 30 seconds. Tip in the diced veg and stir to combine. Add the oregano and half the nutmeg with the tomatoes and basil. Bring to a simmer then cook on a low heat for 30 minutes to thicken, stirring occasionally.

Add the butter, flour and milk to another saucepan, place over a medium heat and whisk constantly until the butter melts and the sauce starts to thicken. Cook for another 5 minutes then season to taste, adding the rest of the nutmeg.

Add a third of the mince to the lasagne dish, followed by a third of the squash slices and a third of the white sauce. Repeat twice more, finishing with a layer of white sauce. Cook for 30–35 minutes, until golden brown and the edges are bubbling nicely. Serve with a salad.

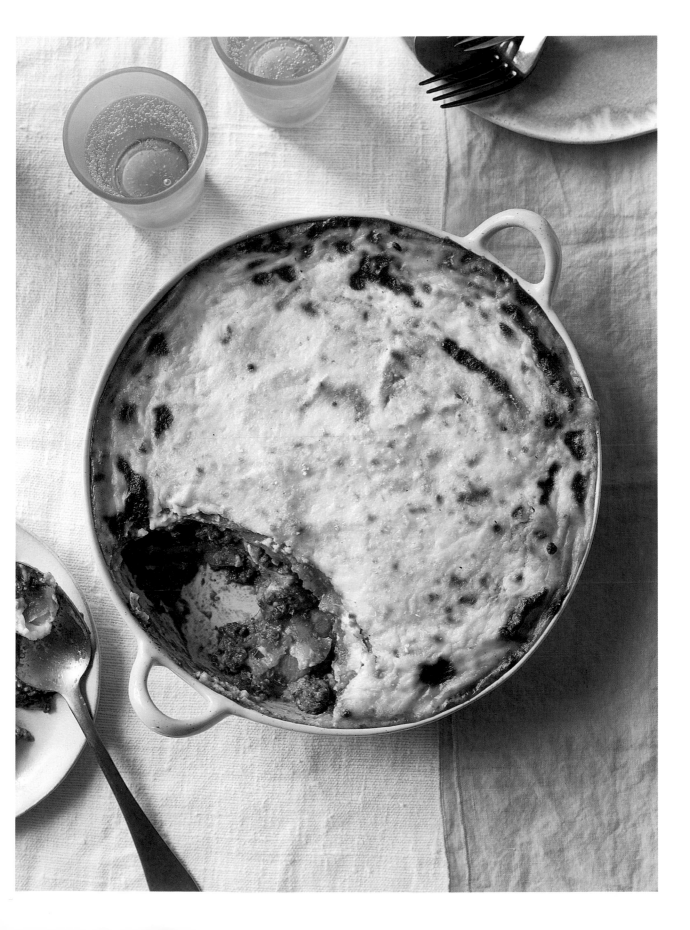

# lamb meatballs with creamy polenta

GOOD FOR
entertaining

This is a real crowd-pleaser. I've been cooking meatballs for years. When I was younger it always made me chuffed when I would learn how to make something that others just shop bought. Essentially with meatballs all you do is place several ingredients into a bowl, mix it and shape into balls. It's very fuss free.

## serves 4

100g breadcrumbs
120ml skimmed milk
500g lamb mince
2 garlic cloves, crushed to a paste
1 tbsp dried oregano
1 tbsp dried basil
500g cherry tomatoes, halved
100g baby spinach
salt and black pepper

### for the polenta
700ml skimmed milk
400ml water
180g quick-cook/instant polenta
40g butter
1 tsp freshly ground nutmeg
30g Parmesan, finely grated

### to serve
basil leaves
Parmesan shavings

Preheat your oven to 200°C/180°C fan/gas 6.

Soak the breadcrumbs in the milk for 5 minutes. Place the lamb mince in a large mixing bowl along with the garlic, oregano, basil and some salt and pepper. Squeeze any excess milk out of the breadcrumbs and add them to the mince.

Use your hands to knead everything altogether into a smooth, even mixture. Shape the mixture into 12 small balls, placing them in a roasting tin as you go.

Put the tin into the hot oven and cook for 15 minutes, then remove the tray, turn the meatballs over and add the tomatoes. Return to the oven for another 15 minutes.

While the meatballs are finishing off, start the polenta. Put the milk and water into a large saucepan and bring to the boil. Once it is boiling, slowly add the polenta in a steady stream, stirring all the time with a wooden spoon. Cook for around 2–3 minutes until the polenta is soft and coming away from the sides of the pan.

Remove from the heat and stir in the butter and nutmeg, then fold through the Parmesan and a little seasoning.

Take a large serving plate and spread the polenta out over the base. Add the baby spinach to the meatballs and tomatoes in the hot tin and stir through until wilted. Spoon on top of the polenta, sprinkle with basil leaves and Parmesan shavings and serve immediately.

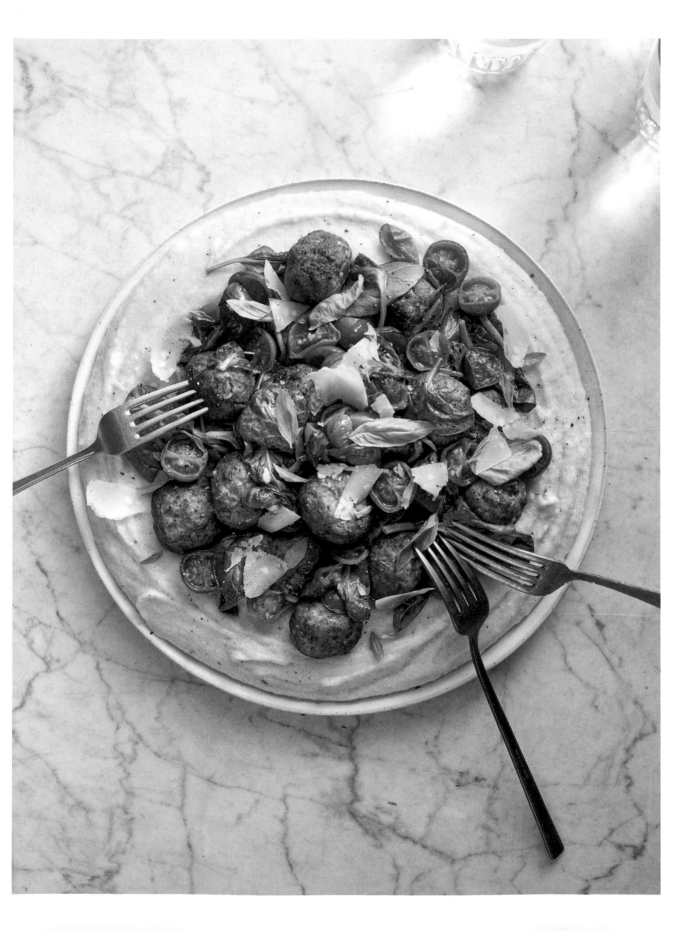

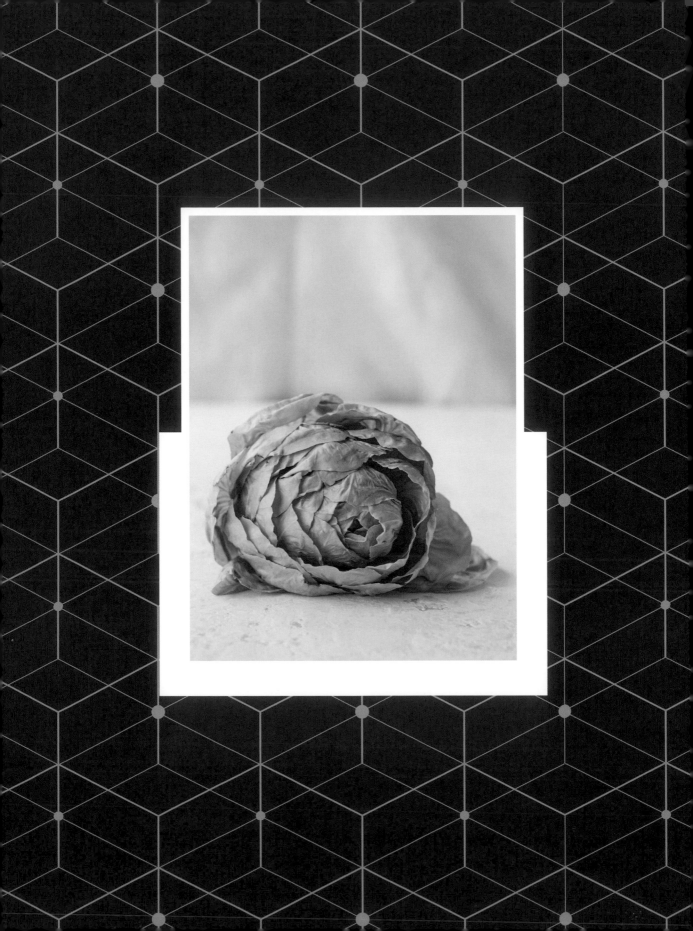

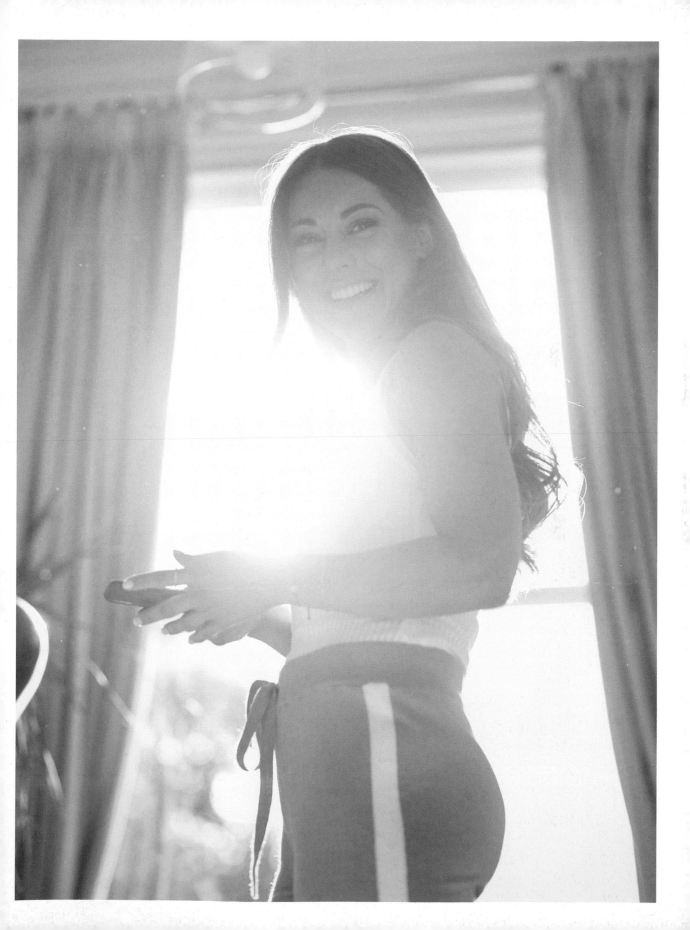

# easy spicy chicken thighs & colourful veg tray bake

My brother Sam is obsessed with chicken thighs so this recipe is dedicated to him. My dad was the first one to encourage us to cook with them and when Sam and I moved into our own house in London he would bring them round from the butcher to cook on the barbecue. We had them all summer long. Not only are they cheaper than other cuts, but are extremely tender and flavoursome when cooked well.

## serves 2

4 large bone-in, skinless chicken thighs
1 tbsp sweet smoked paprika
1 tbsp dried oregano
2 red chillies, chopped
2 garlic cloves, chopped
1 tbsp olive oil
2 orange peppers, deseeded and cut into chunks
6 purple sprouting broccoli florets
½ courgette, cut into chunks
6 radishes, halved
1 tbsp chipotle chilli flakes

Preheat your oven to 200°C/180°C fan/gas 6.

Place the chicken thighs in a large roasting tin.

Put the smoked paprika, oregano, chillies, garlic and olive oil into a mini-chopper and blitz everything together into a paste. Tip this over the chicken and use your hands to rub it all over the thighs.

Add the peppers and broccoli to the roasting tin around the chicken then put into the oven for 20 minutes.

Remove the tin and turn the veg in all the juices. Add the courgette and radishes and return to the oven for another 15–20 minutes.

Remove from the oven and divide everything between two plates. Drizzle over the roasting tin juices and scatter over a few chipotle chilli flakes to add a little smoky heat to the finished dish.

⟨ TIP ⟩
**A lot of my cooking is done in one roasting tin – I call these one-tray wonders!**

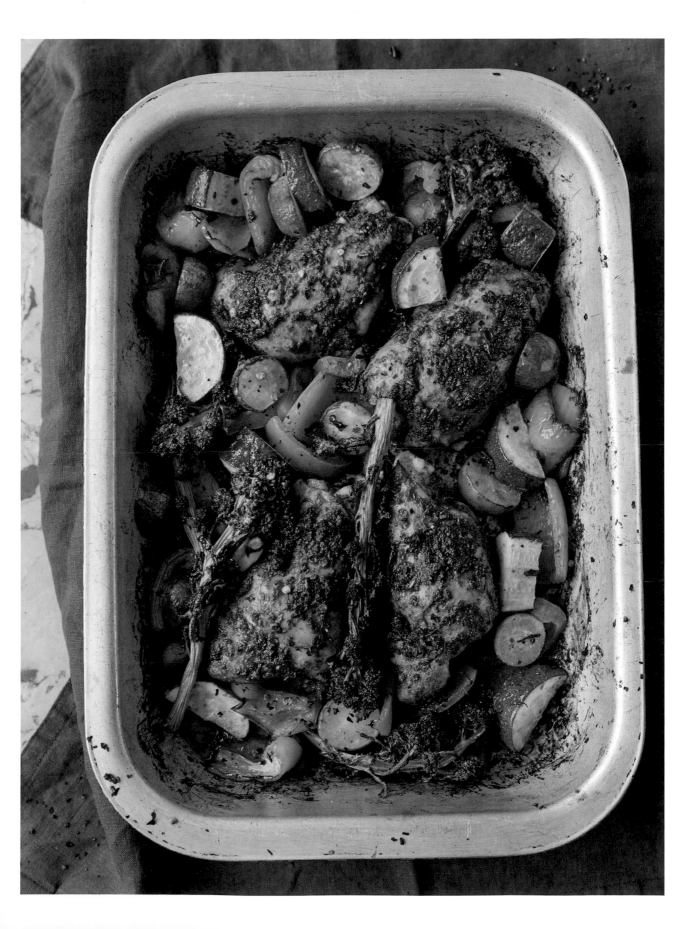

# stuffed baked aubergines

I always felt sorry for vegetarians at dinner parties because they would be served this sort of thing time and time again. When I finally decided to make my own version, I stopped feeling sorry for them! It's delicious! It is worthwhile learning how to perfect cooking rice because it will be useful for the rest of your life – I follow the 'two cups of water to every cup of rice' rule.

## serves 2

2 small aubergines

2 tsp olive oil

1 red onion, chopped

3 garlic cloves, finely grated

1 tbsp tomato purée

1 tsp ground cinnamon

¼ tsp freshly grated nutmeg

1 tbsp dried chilli flakes

1 x 400g tin chopped tomatoes

1 tbsp chopped parsley

1 tsp chopped dill

80g cooked brown rice (about 30g uncooked)

a handful of fresh breadcrumbs

salt and black pepper

fresh herbs, such as parsley, dill and coriander, to serve

Preheat your oven to 220°C/200°C fan/gas 7 and line a roasting tin with non-stick baking paper.

Take the two aubergines and, using a sharp knife, make a long, deep slit down the length of each, being careful not to go fully through. Place them slit side up in the roasting dish and drizzle half the olive oil over them. Put them into the hot oven to roast for 40 minutes.

While the aubergines are roasting, make the filling. Heat the remaining oil in a large saucepan and add the red onion. Cook for 5 minutes over a low heat so it softens but doesn't take on too much colour.

Add the garlic, tomato purée, cinnamon, nutmeg and chilli flakes. Stir everything well and cook for another minute before adding the chopped tomatoes. Turn the heat right down and simmer the sauce for 20 minutes, stirring occasionally.

Once the aubergines have had their time, the flesh should be really soft. Gently open them up down the incision and use a spoon to scrape most of the flesh out, leaving the empty skins intact in the tray. Add the aubergine flesh to the tomato mix and stir to incorporate. Add the parsley, dill and cooked rice, along with some salt and pepper to taste. Cook for 3 minutes.

Remove the filling from the heat and then fill the aubergine skins with the mix. If there's any extra, just add it to the tin. Top the aubergines with the breadcrumbs. Return the tin to the oven, reducing the temperature to 190°C/170°C fan/gas 5 and bake for 20 minutes.

When they are done, serve one aubergine per person and top with fresh herbs.

# brown rice mushroom risotto with crispy sage leaves

Here is my creamy 'sort of healthy' brown rice risotto recipe. Every time I read the ingredients that go into this dish my mouth instantly starts watering. It is pure indulgence with the mixture of crunchy asparagus tips, yummy Parmesan and crisp sage leaves on top.

**serves 2**

## for the risotto

½ tbsp olive oil
1 onion, finely chopped
2 garlic cloves, finely grated
4 sage leaves, roughly chopped
150g easy-cook brown rice
120ml white wine (optional)
400ml vegetable stock
100g chestnut mushrooms, sliced
8 asparagus tips
15g butter
20g Parmesan, grated
salt and black pepper

## for the topping

1 tbsp olive oil
10 sage leaves
10g Parmesan shavings

Preheat your oven to 180°C/160°C fan/gas 4.

Heat the olive oil for the risotto in a flameproof casserole (which has a lid) on a medium heat. Add the onion and cook for 5 minutes to soften. Add the garlic and sage and cook for another 30 seconds.

Add the rice and stir well for about 1–2 minutes, to coat the grains in all the flavour and to heat them. (As with a traditional risotto you want the grains to get nice and hot before you add the liquid.) Add the wine, if using, and cook until it has all but evaporated.

Add the stock, give it all a good stir and take off the heat. Pop the lid on and transfer it to the hot oven for 40 minutes.

About 10 minutes before the end of the cooking time, heat the olive oil for the topping in a frying pan, and add the sage leaves. Cook until crisp then carefully lift out onto some kitchen paper, leaving as much oil as possible behind in the pan. Keep to one side.

Add the mushrooms and asparagus tips to the sage-flavoured oil and turn the heat up. Cook for 4–5 minutes until the mushrooms are golden brown and the asparagus is al dente. Remove from the pan and set aside together.

Remove the casserole from the oven and take the lid off. Stir in the butter and grated Parmesan. Add the mushrooms and asparagus and stir everything together well. Season well with salt and pepper. Divide between two bowls and top with the crispy sage leaves and Parmesan shavings.

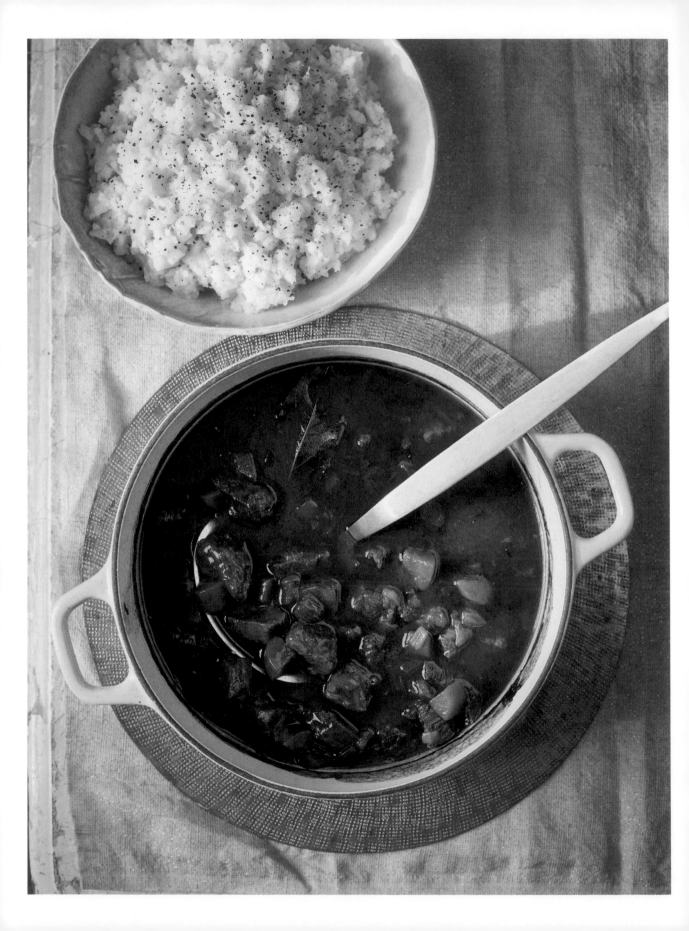

# slow-cooked beef casserole with celeriac & parsnip mash

GOOD FOR
entertaining

Everyone needs a beef casserole recipe in their life and I guarantee you'll find yourself going back to this recipe time and time again. Casseroles and slow-cooked meals lend themselves well to cheaper cuts of meat because the length of cooking time tenderises the meat leaving it soft and succulent.

## serves 4

1 tbsp olive oil

1 onion, diced

2 celery sticks, chopped

2 carrots, peeled and chopped

2 bay leaves

3 sprigs of thyme

2 tbsp brown rice flour

1 tbsp tomato purée

2 tbsp Worcestershire sauce

1 litre beef stock

750g lean diced braising steak

salt and black pepper

### for the mash

1 celeriac (about 500g), peeled and
   cut into 1cm pieces

3 large parsnips (about 300g),
   peeled and cut into 1cm pieces

15g butter

〈 TIP 〉
**This mash is more nourishing than regular mashed potatoes and counts towards your 5-a-day!**

Preheat your oven to 180°C/160°C fan/gas 4 and place a large flameproof casserole over a medium heat. Add the olive oil, onion, celery and carrots. Cook gently for around 10 minutes until everything is softening and turning golden. Add the herbs, flour and tomato purée. Stir to coat the vegetables and cook for 1 minute.

Add the Worcestershire sauce and then slowly add the beef stock, stirring with each addition so that you don't end up with any lumps.

Add the diced beef to the casserole and bring the liquid up to simmering point. If the liquid doesn't quite cover the meat, then top up with a little water. Put the lid on the casserole and transfer to the preheated oven.

Cook for 1 hour, then remove from the oven, give it a stir and return to the oven for another 1 hour. Remove the lid and cook in the oven for a final 30 minutes, then season to taste.

At this point, place the celeriac and parsnips in a large saucepan and cover with cold water and a pinch of salt. Place over a high heat and bring to the boil. Cook for 20 minutes, or until all the veg is really tender. Drain and allow to steam for a couple of minutes to remove excess water.

Return the celeriac and parsnip to the saucepan and add the butter. Mash everything together, with salt and pepper to taste.

# baked sweet potatoes with bean chilli, guacamole & greek yoghurt

A baked potato brings me right back to my school days – however, my version with bean chilli and guacamole is far more sumptuous. I make tonnes of chilli and guacamole to eat with pasta or rice, as a dip or with whatever I fancy for the days following (sometimes straight out of the fridge with a spoon...).

## serves 4

4 large sweet potatoes
½ tbsp olive oil

### for the bean chilli

2 tsp olive oil
1 red onion, diced
2 green chillies, chopped
2 garlic cloves, finely grated
1 tbsp dried oregano
1 tsp ground cinnamon
1 tbsp tomato purée
1 x 400g tin kidney beans, drained
1 x 400g tin borlotti beans, drained
1 x 400g tin chopped tomatoes
1 espresso shot
2 tbsp chopped coriander, plus extra
  leaves to serve

### for the guacamole

2 avocados, roughly chopped
1 small onion, finely chopped
1 red chilli, finely chopped
  juice of 2 limes
2 tbsp finely chopped coriander
salt and black pepper

### to serve

4 tbsp Greek yoghurt
2 jalapeños, thinly sliced

Heat the oil for the chilli in a flameproof casserole. Add the onion and chillies. Cook for a few minutes until the onion starts to look a little translucent, then add the garlic. Cook for 30 seconds to become aromatic then add the oregano, cinnamon and tomato purée. Stir everything well to coat the onion in all the spices.

Add all the beans, the chopped tomatoes, espresso shot and half a bean tin of water. Bring everything up to the boil and then simmer, stirring often.

Preheat your oven to 190°C/170°C fan/gas 5 and scrub the sweet potatoes to make sure the skins are nice and clean. Pat them dry, rub the olive oil over the skins and place them on a baking sheet.

Once the oven is hot, put the potatoes in and bake for 30–35 minutes or until they are soft all the way through; you can test this with a skewer or sharp knife.

While the chilli thickens and the potatoes finish baking, make the guacamole. Using the back of a fork, mash together the avocados, onion, chilli and lime juice in a mixing bowl. Stir through the coriander and a little seasoning.

Add the coriander to the chilli just before serving and check the seasoning – add a little salt and pepper if you like.

Cut the sweet potatoes lengthways and pull them apart. Fill the gap with the bean chilli, top with some guacamole, a dollop of Greek yoghurt, sliced jalapeños and some coriander.

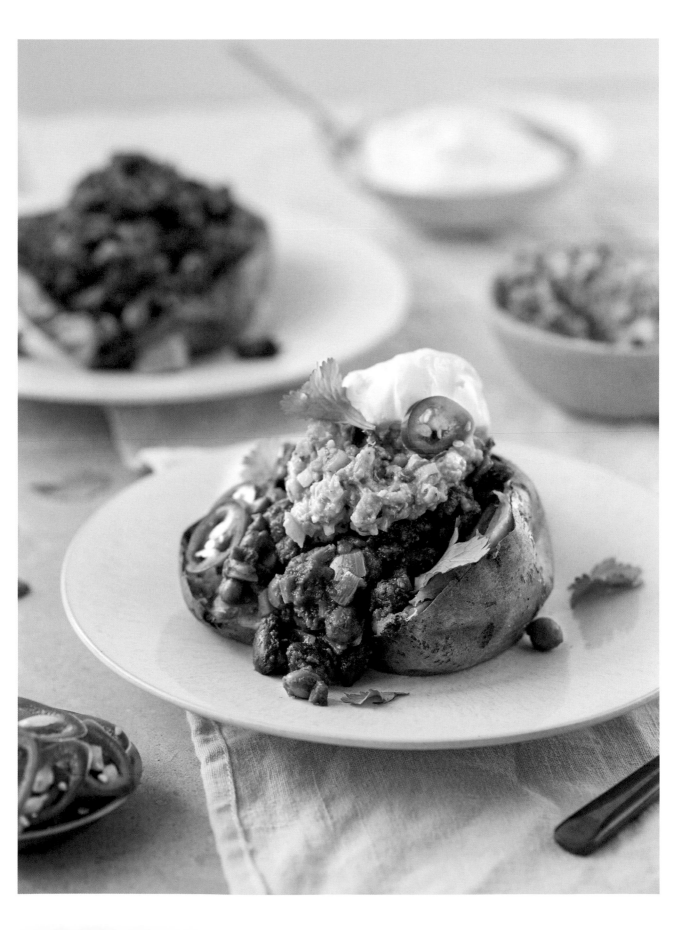

# easy flatbread pizzas

Thick crust, greasy pizzas are something I rarely eat these days; it's great news that I actually way prefer a super crispy thin crust version, adorned with yummy toppings. My pizzas are simple to make, just add ingredients on top to suit your taste buds.

## serves 2

### for the dough

140g spelt flour
a pinch of salt
65–80ml water
½ tsp olive oil

### for the topping suggestions (for 1 pizza)

**prosciutto & sun-dried tomato**

1 tsp sun-dried tomato pesto
¼ mozzarella ball, torn into pieces
40g prosciutto, torn into strips
a handful of basil leaves

**red pepper, courgette & mushroom**

1 tsp sun-dried tomato pesto
½ red pepper, thinly sliced
½ courgette, thinly sliced
3 mushrooms, sliced
¼ mozzarella ball, torn into pieces
a handful of rocket leaves

**spicy chicken & red pepper**

1 tsp basil pesto
½ red pepper, thinly sliced
½ cooked chicken breast, shredded
1 tsp dried chilli flakes
¼ mozzarella ball, torn into pieces

Start by making your dough. If you don't have time to make your own, a bought flatbread will do.

Place the flour in a mixing bowl along with the salt. Use your hand to mix them together, then add enough water to bring the flours together into a rough dough. You don't want it too wet or too dry – it shouldn't be sticky or crumbly.

Pull the dough together, place on your work surface and start to knead. It should become smooth and elastic in around 5–6 minutes of good, strong kneading. If it is at all crumbly, just run your fingers under the tap and continue kneading; if it is too sticky, dust your hands in flour and continue kneading.

Shape the dough into a ball and cover. Allow it to rest for around 10 minutes.

Divide the dough into two pieces and, taking one at a time, shape it into a ball. Then use a rolling pin to roll the dough out into a round approximately 2mm thick.

Heat a large ovenproof frying pan and preheat your grill to its hottest setting. Brush one side of the dough with a little olive oil and place oiled side down in the frying pan. Being careful of the hot pan, assemble your pizza in the frying pan. Use a spoon to spread out the pesto, add the toppings and then take the pan from the hob top and place it under the grill. Cook until the cheese has melted and the bread is cooked through. This whole process should take no more than 5 minutes! Repeat with the second round of dough.

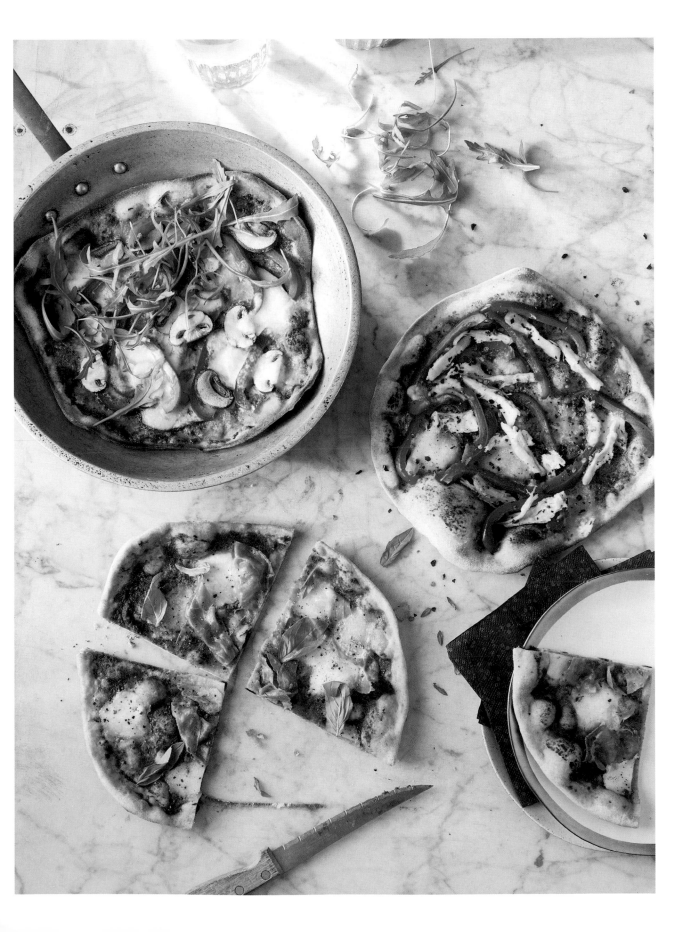

# chicken donburi

GOOD FOR
**post-
workout**

Donburi is quintessential Japanese comfort food. The base layer is a basic sushi rice bowl but then what sits on top can consist of any variety of meat and vegetables. This chicken recipe is a very well-balanced combination that might not be a typical way of presenting food, but I think it is good to try new things.

## serves 2

4 boneless, skinless chicken thighs

1 lemongrass stalk, outer layers removed then roughly chopped

2 garlic cloves, roughly chopped

2cm piece of ginger, roughly chopped

3 spring onions, roughly chopped

juice of ½ lime

1 tbsp light olive oil

200g sushi rice

320ml water

6 broccoli florets, halved

2 tbsp rice wine vinegar

2 tbsp teriyaki sauce

50g pea shoots

1 carrot, peeled and julienned

10g pickled ginger

### to garnish

2 spring onions, shredded

2 tsp sesame seeds

1 tsp dried chilli flakes

< TIP >
**You can add a fried egg for added richness.**

Place the chicken thighs in a shallow dish. Put the lemongrass, garlic, ginger, spring onions, lime juice and olive oil into a mini-chopper and blitz to a paste. Tip this over the chicken thighs and rub it all over them. Leave the chicken in the fridge to marinate for at least 30 minutes.

Preheat your oven to 220°C/200°C fan/gas 7 and line a roasting tin with non-stick baking paper.

Take the chicken out the fridge and put the thighs into the roasting tin and into the oven for 20 minutes.

Put the rice into a saucepan and cover with the water. Bring to the boil, then reduce to a simmer and cook for 10 minutes with a lid on the pan. Remove from the heat and set aside still with the lid on – don't be tempted to peep at it – for another 10–15 minutes.

Bring a small pan of water to the boil and add the broccoli florets. Cook for 3–4 minutes until al dente then drain.

Take the lid off the rice and sprinkle over the rice wine vinegar, then stir to mix.

Once the chicken has had its first 20 minutes, take the tin out and brush the thighs with the teriyaki sauce. Pop them back into the oven for a further 5–6 minutes then remove from the oven, slice into strips and keep handy.

Divide the rice between two bowls. Top the rice with the chicken slices and arrange the broccoli, pea shoots, carrot and pickled ginger around chicken. Sprinkle over the shredded spring onion, sesame seeds and chilli flakes and eat straight away.

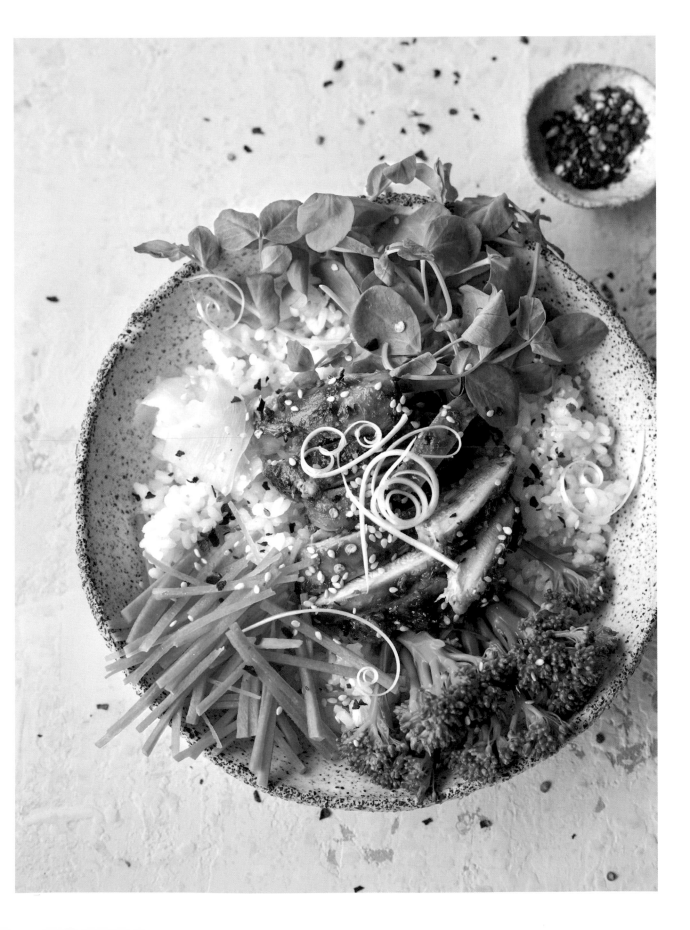

# rack of lamb with braised red cabbage & crunchy rosemary roasties

One of the best parts of growing up was coming home to the smell of my dad's legendary Sunday roasts cooking in the oven. I'm thrilled to share one of my all-time faves with you guys. Few things beat a crispy spud! In my opinion this is one of the most appetising collections of food on one plate EVER. (See next page for photograph.)

## serves 6

2 racks of lamb (about 12–18 ribs, so 2–3 per person)
2 tsp garlic powder
salt and black pepper

### for the braised cabbage

2 tsp olive oil
1 cinnamon stick
3 bay leaves
1 red cabbage, shredded
1 red onion, thinly sliced
50ml red wine vinegar
100ml water
20g unsalted butter, cubed

### for the rosemary potatoes

2kg Maris Piper potatoes, peeled and cut into chunks
3 tbsp olive oil
6 sprigs of rosemary

Start with the cabbage as this is going to take the longest to cook. Heat the olive oil in a large flameproof casserole on a medium heat and add the cinnamon and bay leaves. Add the cabbage and onion and sprinkle over the red wine vinegar. Add the water and give everything a good stir. Drop the cubes of butter over the top and put the lid on. Turn the heat right down and cook for 30 minutes, then take the lid off and give it a good stir. Repeat this once more before starting the potatoes. Then repeat until you are ready to serve, so that it gently cooks for a total of around 2–2½ hours.

Preheat your oven to 220°C/200°C fan/gas 7.

Put the potato chunks into a large saucepan and cover with cold water and a generous pinch of salt. Put the pan on a high heat, bring to the boil and cook the potatoes for 12–14 minutes until just soft through and the edges just starting to break down.

While the potatoes are boiling, put the olive oil into a roasting tin and put it into the oven to heat up. Once the potatoes are done, drain them and allow to steam dry in a colander for a couple of minutes.

Take the roasting tin out of the oven and, very carefully as the oil will be very hot, tip the potatoes into the oil. Tip the tin to collect the oil in one corner and use a spoon to baste the potatoes. Lay the rosemary sprigs around the potatoes and season with salt and pepper. Return the tray to the oven and roast them for 20 minutes, then take them out, turn them over and return for another 25–30 minutes until golden and crisp.

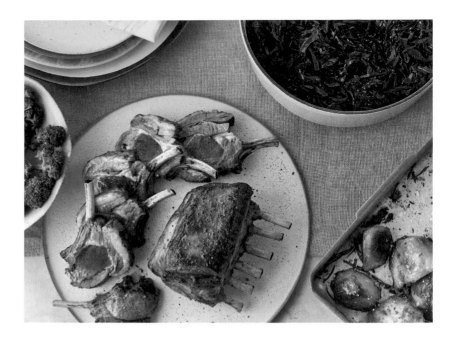

When the potatoes have 25 minutes left, take the racks of lamb and place them on a chopping board. Sprinkle the garlic powder and some salt and pepper over them. Use your hands to rub the seasoning all over them.

Put a large frying pan over a medium–high heat and add the racks, skin side down. Let them cook like this for 3–4 minutes until beautifully browned. Then flip them and seal the meaty underside for around a minute. Lastly seal both ends for a minute and then place them in a roasting tin. Put them into the hot oven with the potatoes, moving the potatoes down to a lower shelf.

Roast the lamb for 12–14 minutes for it to be blushing, then remove and let it rest for 10 minutes. Turn the heat down in the oven and keep the potatoes warm until you are ready to serve.

Carve the lamb into either individual or pairs of chops. Serve alongside the rosemary potatoes and the braised red cabbage, with broccoli if you like.

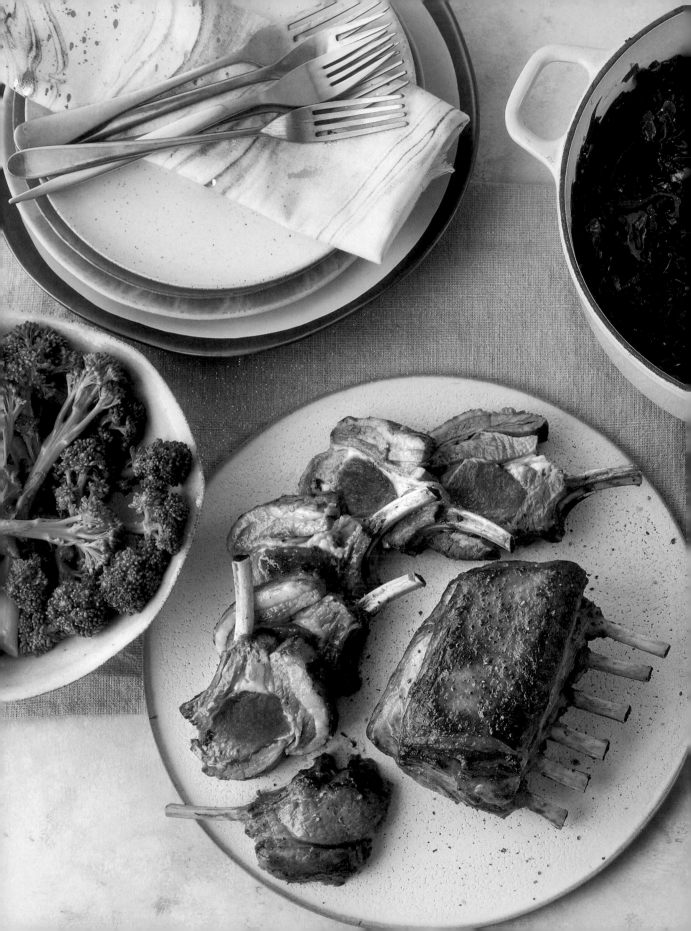

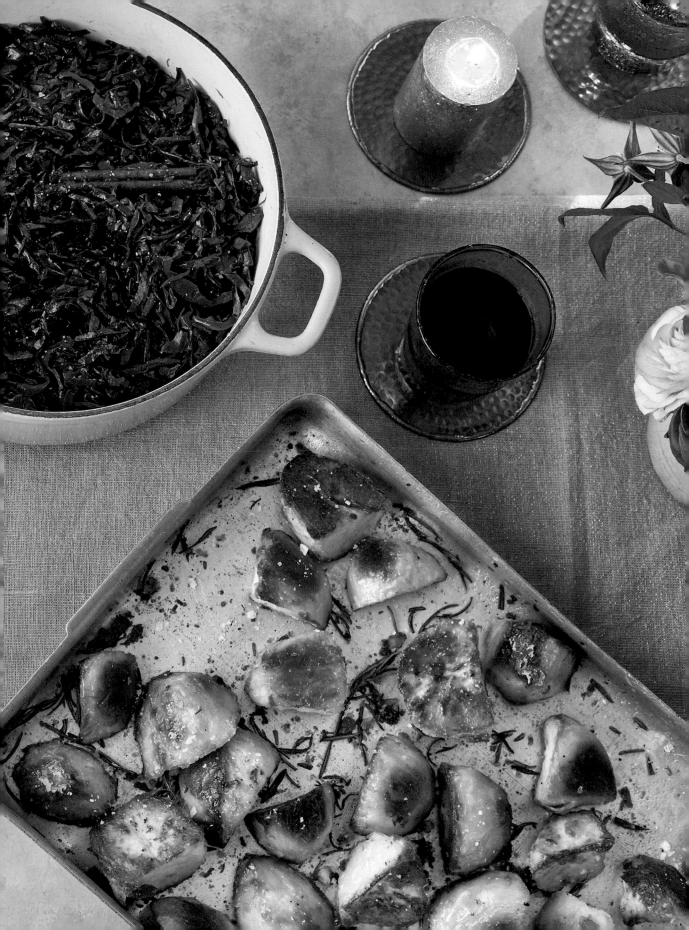

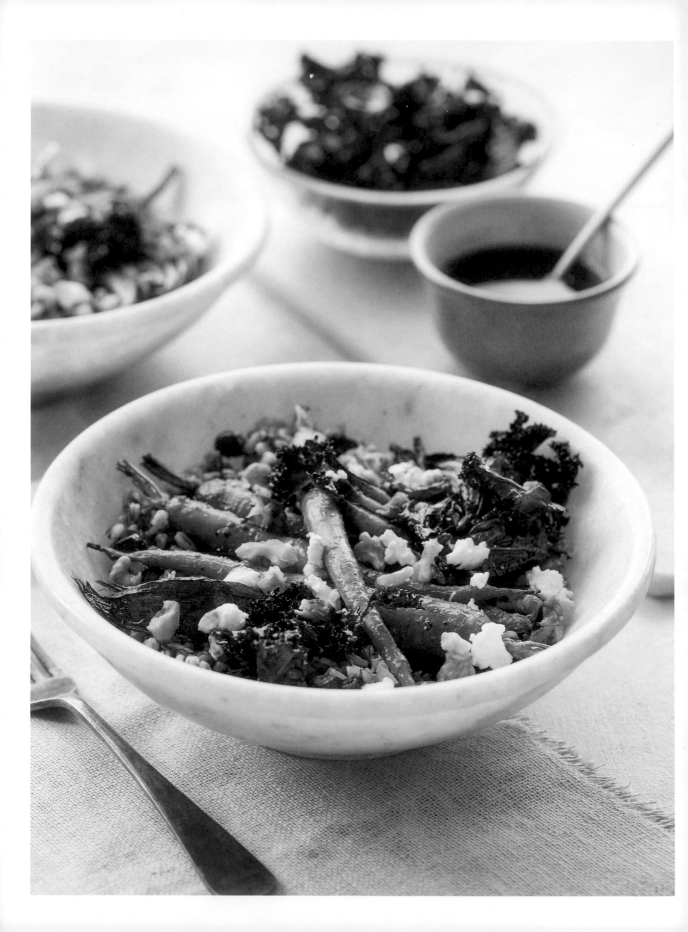

# roasted carrot farro salad with kale, goat's cheese & walnuts

Farro is an ancient wheat grain. Like barley it remains a little chewy when cooked which makes it a brilliant addition to salads. Goat's cheese and walnuts are a classic combo but the addition of roasted carrots and the honey dressing add a subtle sweetness. If you don't want to use farro then you could substitute with a different grain, but the cooking times will vary.

## serves 2

1 tbsp olive oil
180g baby carrots
1 red onion, peeled and cut into
  6 wedges
40g kale, leaves torn and tough
  stalks removed
100g farro
60g pomegranate seeds
1 tbsp roughly chopped coriander
1 tbsp roughly chopped dill
1 tbsp roughly chopped parsley
40g goat's cheese
15g walnuts, roughly chopped
salt and black pepper

### for the dressing
2 tsp rose harissa paste
2 tsp runny honey
2 tsp extra virgin olive oil
juice of 1 lemon

Preheat the oven to 200°C/180°C fan/gas 6 and line a roasting tin with non-stick baking paper.

Add the olive oil, baby carrots, red onion, kale and some salt and pepper. Toss everything together and pop into the oven to roast for 20 minutes.

While that is cooking, place the farro in a saucepan and cover with cold water. Put on a medium–high heat and bring to the boil, then reduce the heat to a simmer and cook the farro for 12 minutes, or until al dente. Drain and transfer to a mixing bowl.

Next, add the pomegranate seeds and chopped herbs to the bowl and mix everything well.

Divide between two serving bowls and top with the roast carrots, onion and crispy kale. Crumble the goat's cheese over the top and sprinkle with the walnuts.

Using a whisk, mix the dressing ingredients in a little bowl, with salt and pepper to taste, and drizzle some over each bowl.

# fish tacos

GOOD FOR
*entertaining*

I remember visiting my best friend when she was studying
Spanish in Merida, which is in the Yucatan peninsula of Mexico.
She taught me the real difference between tacos, fajitas,
burritos, enchiladas etc. A taco is simply meat or fish and
toppings put inside a tortilla. You can use many different kinds
of fish in a fish taco but my preference is monkfish because it is
meaty yet has a light, delicate flavour.

## serves 2

250g monkfish loin (you could use
  cod or another firm white fish)
1 tsp olive oil
½ tsp ground cumin
½ tsp paprika
¼ tsp cayenne pepper
salt and black pepper

### for the quick salsa

½ avocado, diced
2 tomatoes, diced
2 spring onions, chopped
1 tbsp roughly chopped coriander
juice of 1 lime

### for the taco sauce

2 tbsp natural yoghurt
finely grated zest and juice of 1 lime
1 tsp sriracha

### to serve

4 small flatbreads (see page 150 for
  home-made, but instead of making
  2 big ones, make 4 small)
40g red cabbage, shredded
40g white cabbage, shredded
1 red onion, quick-pickled (see page
  118)
coriander leaves
dried chilli flakes *(optional)*

Put the monkfish into a shallow dish and add the olive oil, cumin,
paprika, cayenne and some salt and pepper. Turn the fish over and
over until it's all coated.

Place a frying pan on a high heat and, once hot, lay in the fish. Cook
for 2 minutes each side. Try not to move it before the time is up, so that
you get some charring – this just makes it taste better. Then remove
from the heat and put it on a chopping board to rest – the residual
heat will keep the fish cooking and finish it off.

Making the salsa is as simple as mixing all the ingredients together in a
bowl and seasoning with some salt and pepper.

To make the taco sauce, place everything in a small bowl and whisk
together well.

To serve, cut the monkfish into 5mm slices; take a flatbread and load
it with red and white cabbage, some salsa, monkfish slices, pickled
red onion, taco sauce, coriander leaves, and chilli flakes if you want
it even more fiery!

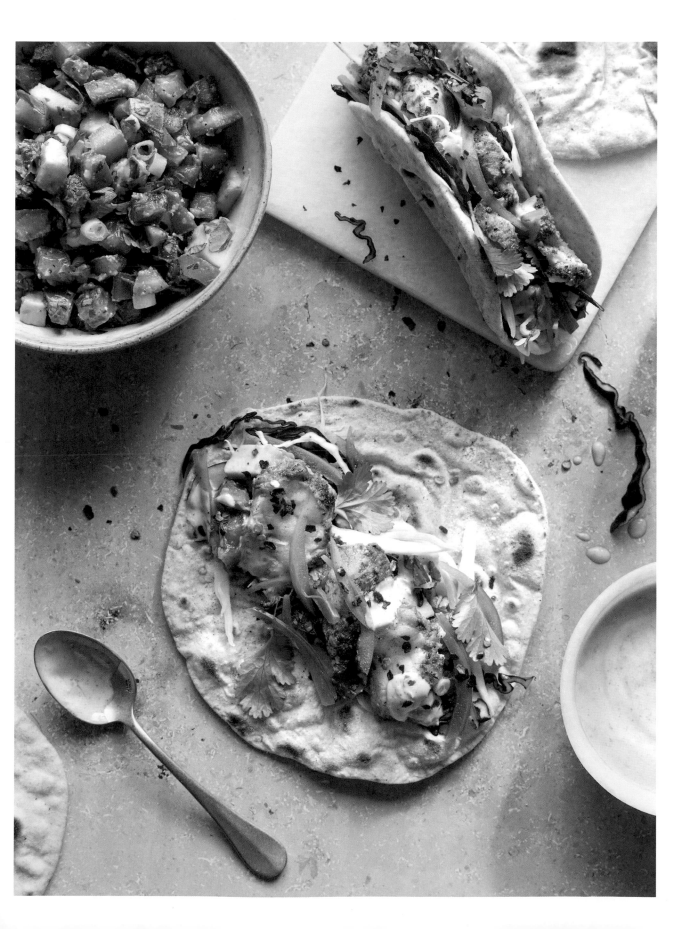

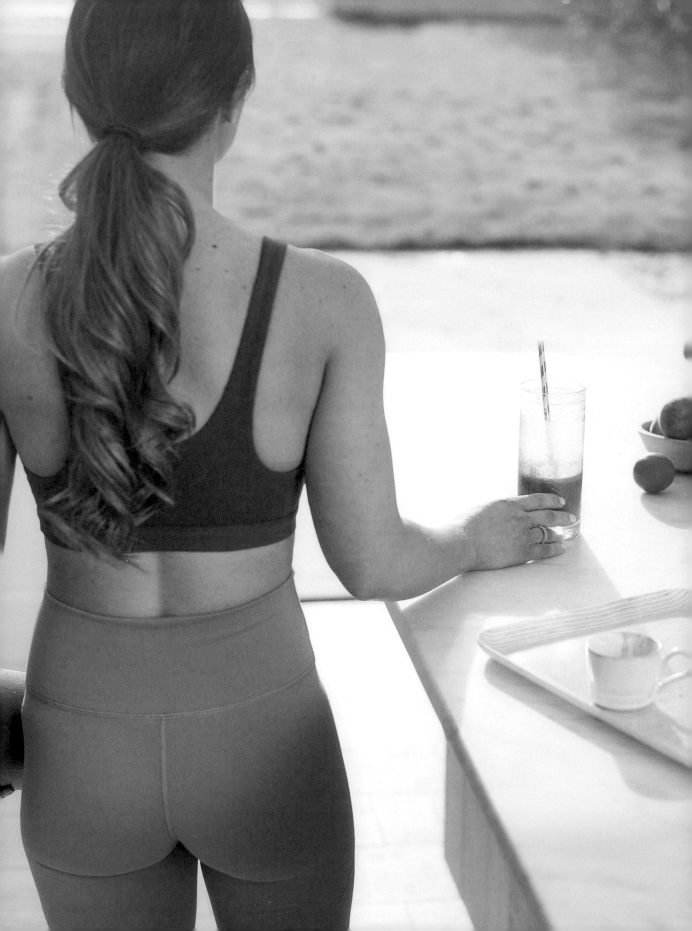

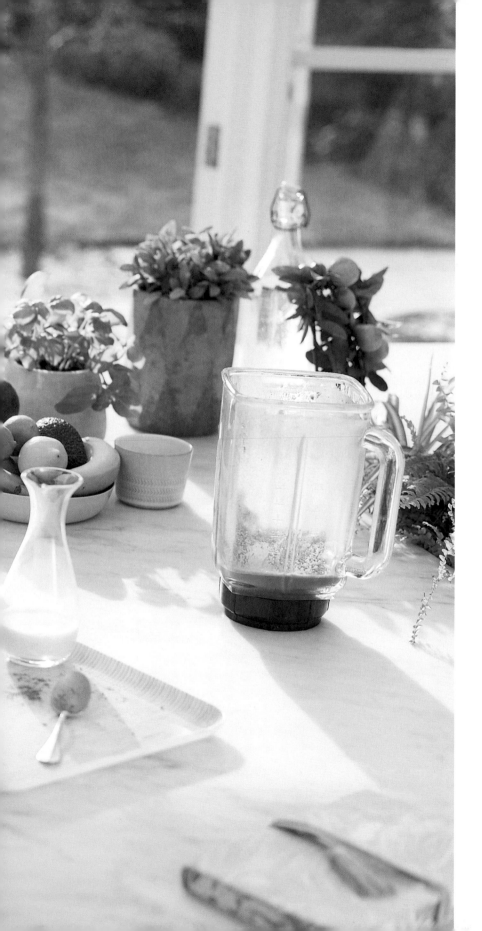

smoothies
& snacks

# smoothies

Smoothies are great because all you have to do is place the ingredients in your blender, top up with liquid, blitz until it is lovely and smooth, then pour out and enjoy. You can add ice if you like a really cold smoothie, but keeping the ingredients in the fridge before you use them will make a cold and refreshing drink. Optional protein boosts include hemp seeds, milled flaxseed, wheat germ, sunflower seeds, chia seeds or good-quality protein powder. Although smoothies retain all the fibre and nutrients of the fruits, they shouldn't be used to replace meals. I enjoy them as a treat on the go or as a pudding. (*See next page for photographs.*)

--- **all serve 1** ---

### banana, yoghurt, honey, ginger

1 banana, sliced
100g fat-free Greek yoghurt
1 tsp runny honey
1cm piece of ginger, finely chopped
150ml almond milk or water
  (more if you like it looser)

### frozen berries, peanut butter, rolled oats

100g frozen red berries
  (strawberries, raspberries,
  redcurrants, blackberries etc.)
1 tsp smooth peanut butter
30g rolled oats
200ml almond milk (more if you like
  it looser)
1 tbsp vanilla protein powder

### almond milk, banana coffee, cocoa

1 tbsp vanilla protein powder
200ml almond milk
1 banana, sliced
1–2 tbsp raw cocoa powder
60ml cold espresso

### peach, banana, carrot

2 peaches, stoned and roughly
  chopped
½ small banana, sliced
1 tbsp vanilla protein powder
1 carrot, grated
250ml almond milk

### green smoothie

60g frozen spinach (or use kale)
40g low-fat Greek yoghurt
½ avocado
1 tsp spirulina (optional – you could
  try starting with ¼ tsp and build up)
300ml coconut water (more if you
  like it looser)

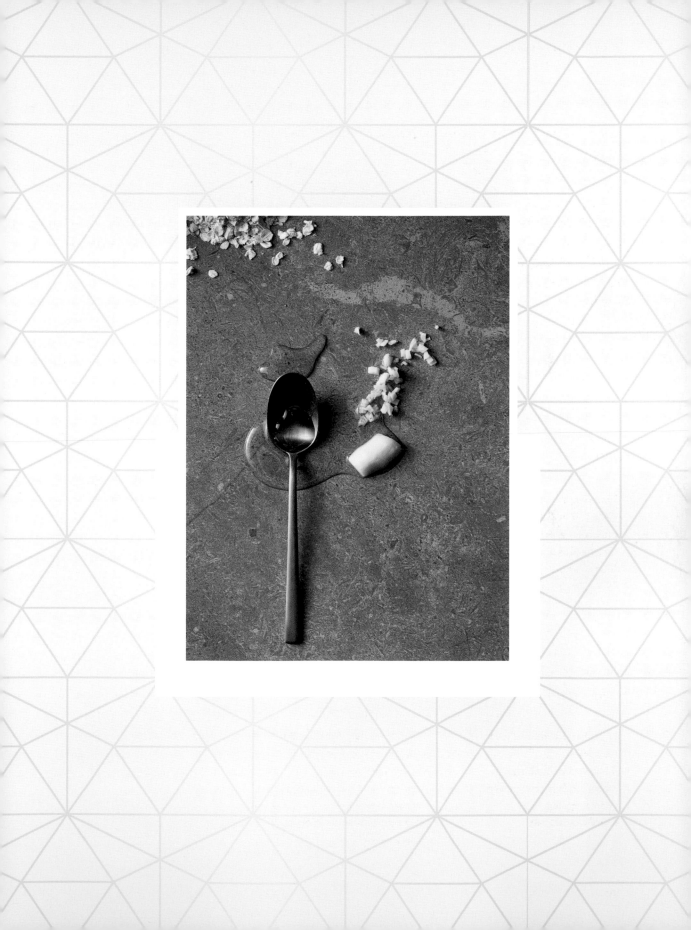

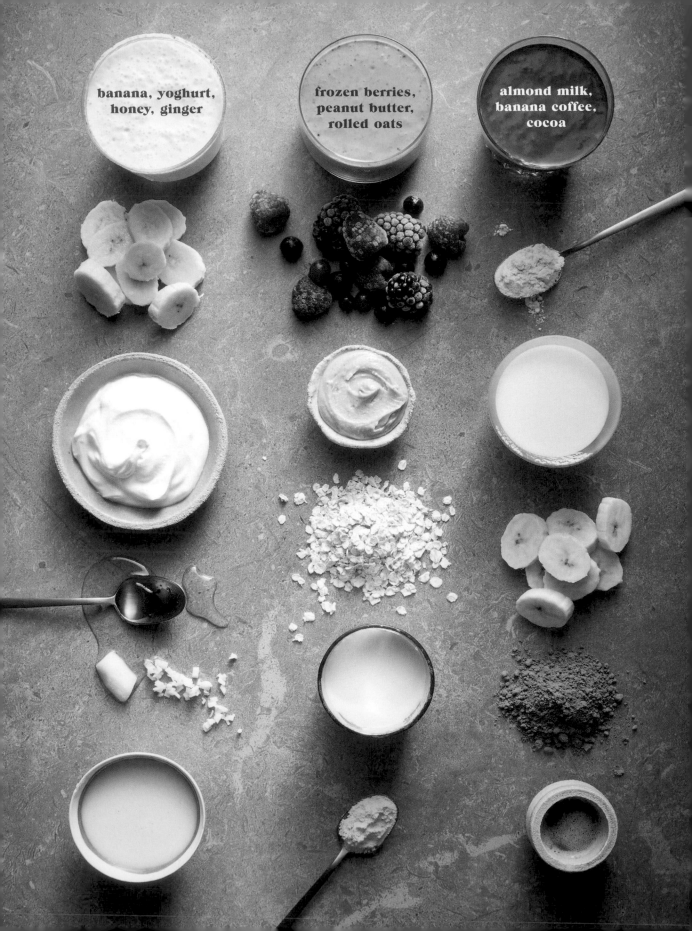

banana, yoghurt,
honey, ginger

frozen berries,
peanut butter,
rolled oats

almond milk,
banana coffee,
cocoa

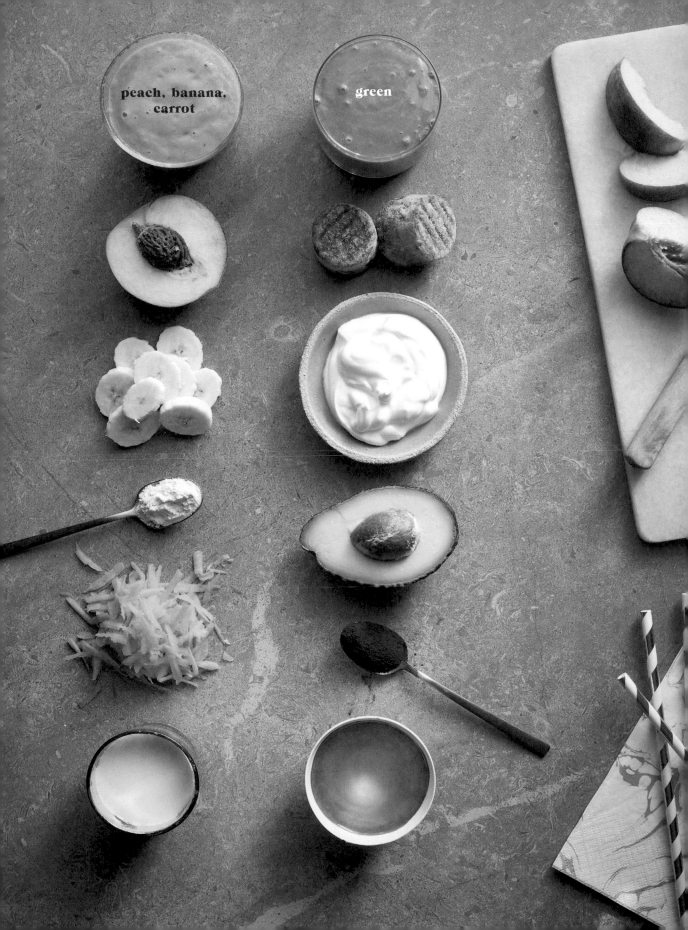

peach, banana, carrot

green

# cinnamon tortillas with strawberry & avocado salsa

This is a quirky take on a typical Mexican favourite. The addition of sweet strawberries to a salsa is massively underrated. Not only does it bring the colour, but the taste and texture is sensational. For even more flavour, include mango in the mix.

**serves 4**

4 spelt flatbreads (see page 150 for home-made)
2 tsp olive oil
½ tsp ground cinnamon

**for the salsa**

1 large avocado, chopped
200g strawberries, chopped
1 red chilli, deseeded and finely chopped
1 tbsp finely chopped mint leaves
juice of 1 lime
a pinch of salt

Preheat your oven to 200°C/180°C fan/gas 6.

Cut each flatbread into 4 pieces and place on two baking sheets.

Mix together the oil and cinnamon and lightly brush one side of the flatbreads with a little of the mix. Pop into the hot oven for around 10 minutes to dry out and crisp up into tortillas.

While they are in the oven, make the salsa by simply placing all the ingredients in a bowl and mixing together.

Serve the salsa alongside the cinnamon tortillas.

< TIP >
**Use heart-shaped cookie cutters to make these low-fat sweet snacks even sweeter**

# blueberry burst slices

These snacks are the perfect way to take you through to your next meal because they are incredibly filling. You can prepare them in batches and keep them to eat over the following week or you can take them to work to share with colleagues and increase your popularity! They are good for breakfast too.

## makes 10 slices

200g blueberries
160g spelt flour
100g ground almonds
40g coconut sugar
1 tsp ground cinnamon
1 tsp baking powder
4 medium eggs
2 tbsp honey
a pinch of salt
50g oats

Preheat your oven to 180°C/160°C fan/gas 4 and line a 20cm square cake tin with non-stick baking paper, making sure the paper comes above the level of the tin (to make lifting it out easier once cooked).

Place 100g of the blueberries in a food processor with the flour, ground almonds, coconut sugar, cinnamon, baking powder, eggs, honey and salt. Blitz until smooth.

Pour out into a mixing bowl and stir through the remaining blueberries and the oats. Don't be deterred by the colour at this point, which is rather an interesting shade of purple – it bakes up really nicely!

Transfer the mixture to your lined cake tin, level it off and pop into the oven to bake for 20–22 minutes, until golden brown. A skewer inserted into the middle will come out clean (except perhaps for a little blueberry juice).

Remove from the oven and allow to cool in the tin for 5 minutes before carefully lifting it out and allowing to cool on a wire rack. Cut into 10 slices and store in an airtight container, somewhere cool, for up to 5 days.

# courgette loaf

I believe that courgette is still pretty underrated. I've started using it in so many aspects of my cooking, from raw salads where it acts like rice noodles soaking up dressing, to soups to cakes. I was gobsmacked the first time my friend presented me with a slice of courgette bread she'd made at home, but I left with the recipe saved on my phone.

## makes 16 slices

2 courgettes, grated (about 220g in total)
140ml olive oil
4 large eggs
2 tsp vanilla extract
200g plain flour
1 tsp baking powder
2 tsp ground cinnamon
a pinch of nutmeg
a pinch of salt
80g toasted walnuts, roughly chopped
80g dark chocolate chips

### for the serving suggestions

- 1 tsp nut butter (I love cashew here)
- butter and 1 tsp jam
- 1 tsp runny honey
- ricotta or another light cream cheese
- a drizzle of extra-virgin olive oil

Preheat the oven to 180°C/160°C fan/gas 4 and line a 900g loaf tin with non-stick baking paper.

Squeeze out as much liquid from the grated courgette as you can – placing it in a clean towel and then wringing it is a great way of doing this. Then place it in a large mixing bowl.

Combine the olive oil with the eggs and vanilla in a jug and beat together well to combine.

Add the flour, baking powder, cinnamon, nutmeg and salt to the courgette and stir to mix. Pour in the egg mixture and stir well to combine, folding everything together.

Lastly, fold in the walnuts and chocolate chips. Pour the batter into the lined loaf tin and level out the top. Bake on the middle shelf of the hot oven for 50–55 minutes.

You'll know it's done when it is golden brown and a skewer inserted into the middle comes out clean. Remove it from the oven and let it cool on a cooling rack for 15 minutes before you turn it out. Allow to cool for another 10 minutes before slicing.

It's absolutely delicious on its own but you could always top it with some nut butter or one of the other serving suggestions.

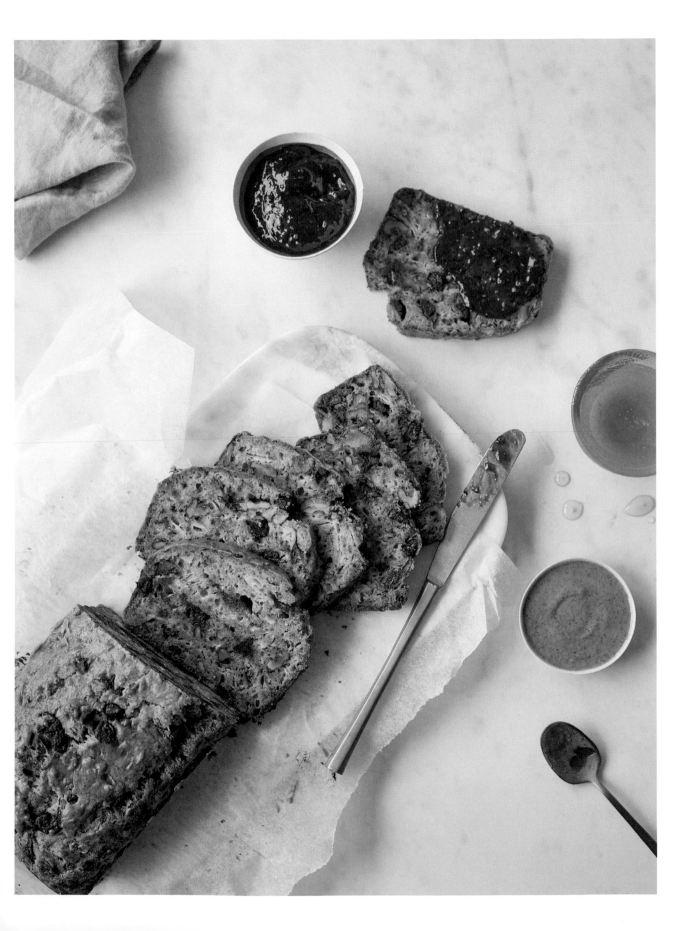

# quinoa, almond & chia seed cookies

Everybody loves a cookie and I believe that we all deserve a little bit of what we love every now and then even if it is in the form of a good old-fashioned biscuit. This is one of my favourite 'healthy' versions of a cookie that I don't believe compromises on flavour. There is no flour, no oil and no added sugar so you won't feel too guilty chowing down on a couple when you take them round to your partner's family for the weekend.

**makes 12**

1 tbsp smooth peanut butter
2 medium eggs
1 medium-sized ripe banana, roughly chopped
150g quinoa flakes
50g ground almonds
50g oats
1½ tsp baking powder
1 tsp ground cinnamon
50g dark chocolate chips
2 tbsp chia seeds

Preheat the oven to 180°C/160°C fan/gas 4 and line a baking sheet with non-stick baking paper.

Put the peanut butter, eggs and banana into a mixing bowl and use electric beaters to whisk everything together until light and foamy.

Fold in the quinoa flakes, ground almonds, oats, baking powder, cinnamon, chocolate chips and chia seeds. Mix together thoroughly and pull everything together into a rough dough.

Divide into 12 equal pieces and roll into balls. Spread them out on the baking tray and flatten them a little with the palm of your hand.

Pop them into the hot oven and bake for 12–14 minutes until golden brown. Leave to cool on the baking sheet for a couple of minutes before transferring to a wire rack to cool completely.

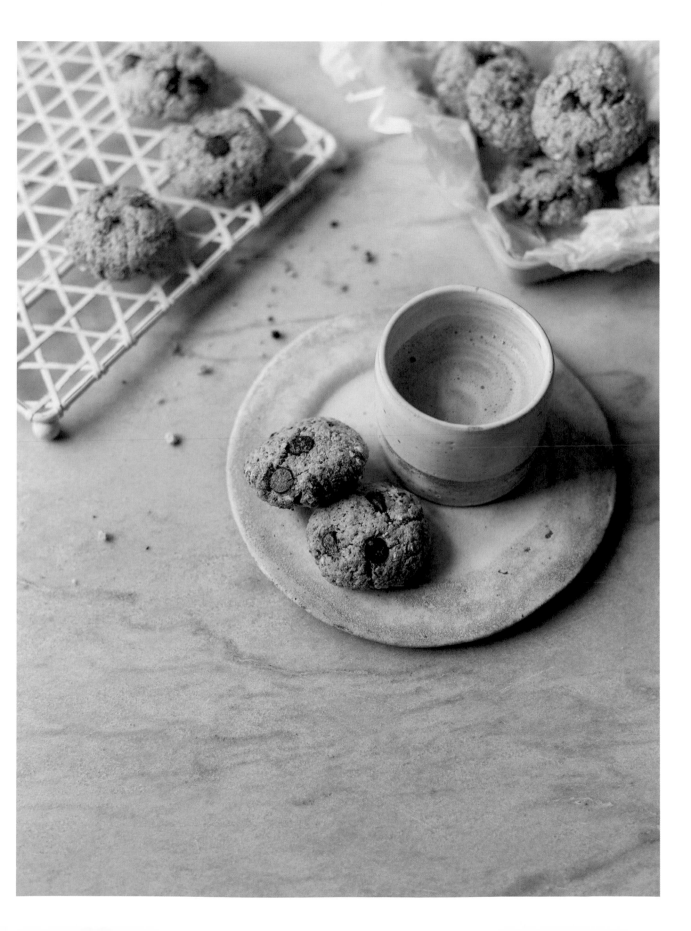

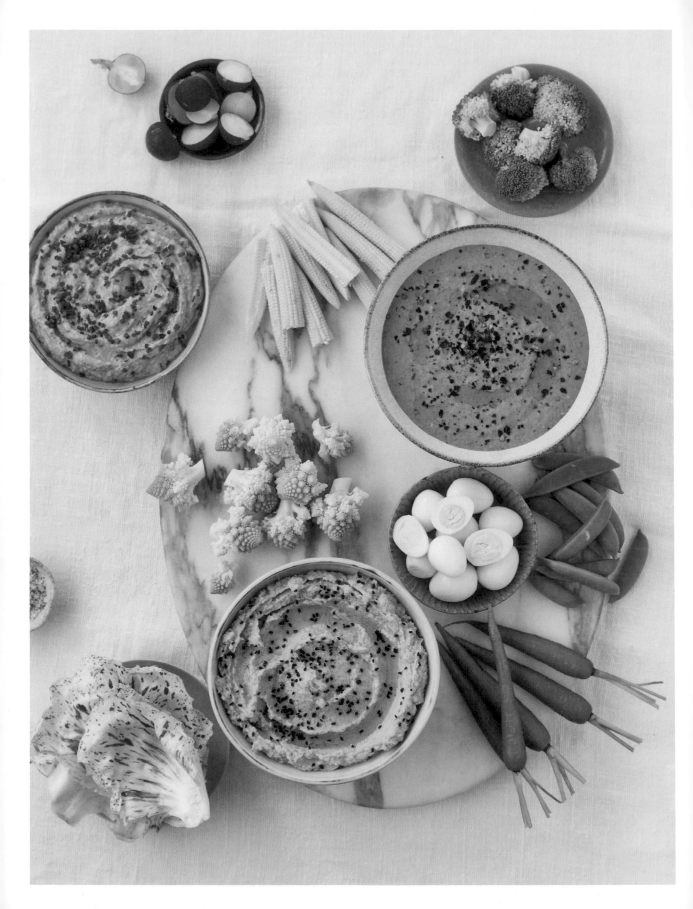

# dips

Crudités for dipping can be anything you fancy! Mix up the colours and textures and include things like green beans, baby corn, broccoli, cauliflowers, different carrots, sliced beetroot, sugar snaps, chicory leaves and radish. A hollowed out large fruit or vegetable can be a fun bowl for serving too.

**all serve 8**

## roast carrot hummus

200g carrots, cut into chunks
1 tbsp olive oil
1 x 400g tin chickpeas, drained
1 small garlic clove, chopped
2 tbsp tahini
juice of 1 lemon
salt and black pepper

### to serve
1 tsp extra virgin olive oil
1 tsp nigella seeds

Preheat the oven to 220°C/ 200°C fan/gas 7. Line a baking sheet with non-stick baking paper. Add the carrots and drizzle over the olive oil and some salt and pepper. Roast in the oven for 20 minutes or until tender all the way through.

Place the carrots in a food processor along with the chickpeas, garlic, tahini and lemon juice. Blitz until smooth. Scrape into a bowl and serve drizzled with extra virgin olive oil and sprinkled with nigella seeds.

## roasted garlic & red pepper

1 bulb of garlic, separated into cloves (left unpeeled)
4 red peppers, deseeded and cut into chunks
1 tbsp olive oil
1 tsp sweet smoked paprika
100g mascarpone
juice of 1 lemon
salt and black pepper

### to serve
1 tsp extra virgin olive oil
1 tsp chipotle chilli flakes

Preheat the oven to 200°C/ 180°C fan/gas 6. Line a baking sheet with non-stick baking paper. Add the garlic and chopped pepper. Drizzle with olive oil and season. Roast for 25 minutes, until the garlic is soft and the peppers are starting to char.

Squeeze the garlic cloves from their skins into a food processor. Add the pepper and cool. Add the rest of the ingredients. Season and blitz until smooth. Scrape into a bowl. Drizzle with oil and sprinkle with chilli flakes.

## green dip
### (avocado, yoghurt, cress, parsley)

2 large avocados, roughly chopped
1 tbsp fat-free Greek yoghurt
4 spring onions, roughly chopped
2 tbsp basil leaves
2 tbsp parsley leaves
grated zest and juice of 1 lemon
1 tbsp extra virgin olive oil
salt and black pepper

### to serve
1 tsp extra virgin olive oil
1 tsp finely chopped chives

Put all the ingredients for the dip in a food processor, with salt and pepper to taste, and blitz until smooth.

Scrape into a bowl and serve with a drizzle of extra virgin olive oil and a sprinkling of chopped chives on top.

# quick pre- & post-workout refuellers

Here are some of my go-to snacks that I eat before or after a workout – these are easy to make but full of goodness. It is worth remembering that what you eat before and after training is important. You need energy beforehand to power you through and then you need protein afterwards to rebuild damaged muscles and carbs to restore your energy stores.

### all serve 2

## avocado & egg toasts

Hard-boil **2 eggs** for 8 minutes. Drain and run under cold water to stop them cooking (you can also boil them in advance and keep them in your fridge for a few days). Once cool, peel them. In a small mixing bowl, mash together **½ avocado, 2 chopped spring onions, the juice from 1 lime** and **½ tsp dried chilli flakes**. Toast **2 slices of sourdough** and top with the mixture. Then quarter the eggs and serve on top. Season to taste.

## yoghurt & protein powder

One of the best inventions ever is the combination of natural **low-fat or fat-free yoghurt** with protein powder. Depending on the flavour of the protein powder, you can create something that tastes better than pudding. I like to mix my yoghurt with **vanilla protein powder** to make a silky smooth bowl that tastes like melted white chocolate. To add texture, throw in some **frozen berries** and a little **granola**.

## rye bread with nut butter & banana

I like to keep plenty of rye – or 'Ryan' bread as we call it at home – in our freezer. When I am pushed for time, I will pop a couple of slices in the toaster and slather them in **peanut butter** with **a sliced banana** on top.

## easy wraps

Something else that I always keep in the fridge are **corn or wholegrain tortilla wraps**. That way, post-workout I can construct a really quick snack by throwing together anything I have lingering in the fridge. My favourite combinations are **tomato, basil** and **mozzarella** (like a caprese salad) with the occasional slice of **salami**. My other go-to is **chicken** with **crunchy lettuce leaf** and **avocado**.

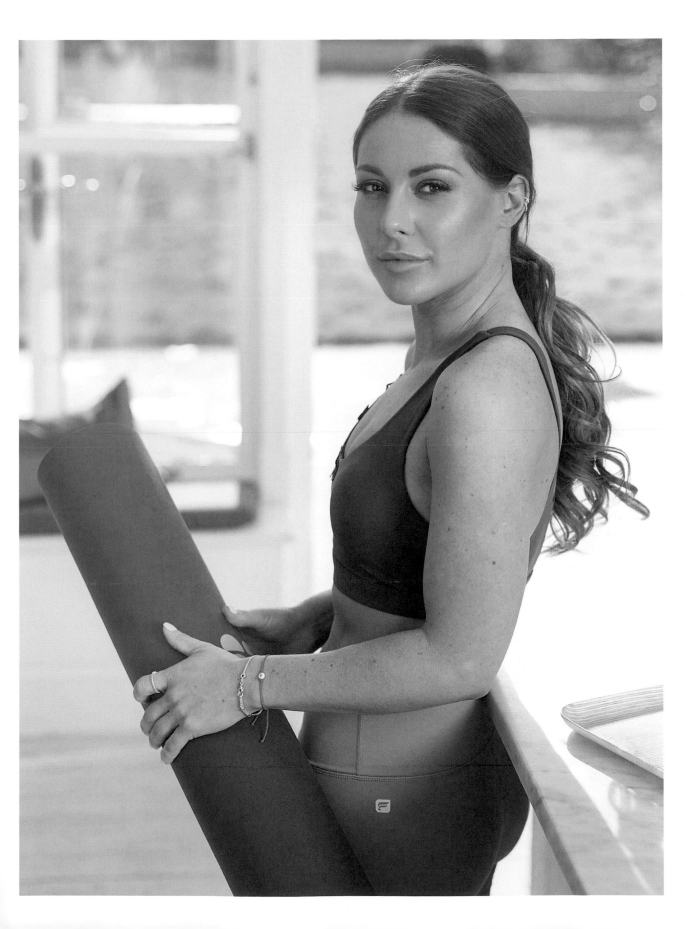

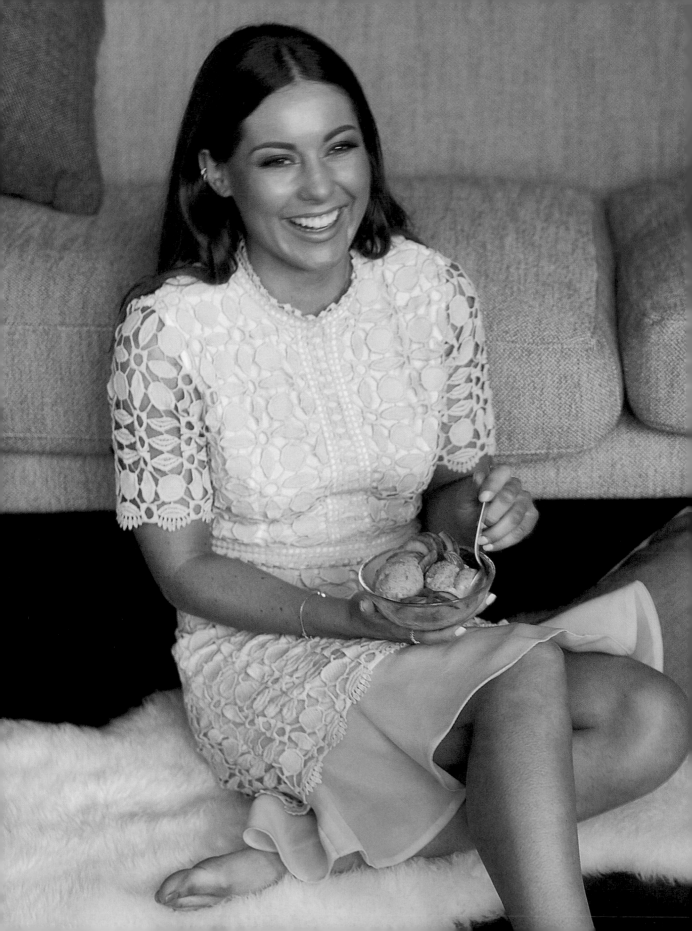

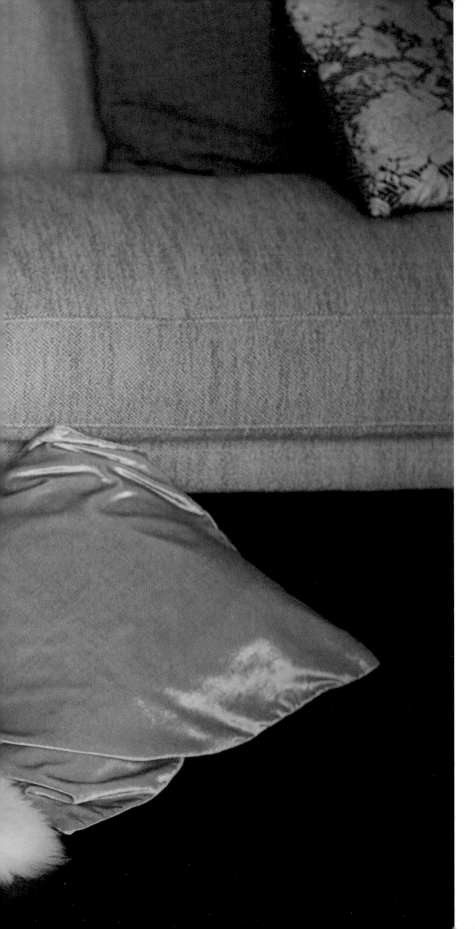

puddings
& treats

# lemon spelt cupcakes

It was necessary for me to include a lemon pudding. I have an obsession with the flavour of lemon in puddings – lemon meringue pie, lemon curd, lemon tart, lemon sorbet, lemon drizzle cake... the list goes on! I decided to give you guys a recipe for a perfectly light and fluffy cupcake rather than a whole cake because I find there is less room for error when making miniatures, plus they are already portioned for you, and they cook even faster. Another bonus is that they are far more fun to decorate.

**makes 12**

150g unsalted butter, softened
150g coconut sugar
3 medium eggs
160g spelt flour
1½ tsp baking powder
finely grated zest and juice of
  2 lemons
80g mascarpone
raspberry or acai berry freeze-dried
sprinkles, to decorate (optional)

> ⟨ TIP ⟩
> **I like to top
> with extra zest.**

Preheat your oven to 180°C/160°C fan/gas 4 and line a cupcake tin with paper cases.

Add the butter and sugar to a large mixing bowl and beat with electric beaters until pale and fluffy. This will take a couple of minutes. Then add one egg at a time, making sure the first one is well mixed in before adding the next.

Add the flour, baking powder and all the lemon zest, but only half the juice (save the rest for the icing).

Beat everything together until combined, then place a spoonful in each of the paper cases. Pop the tin into the oven and bake for 18–20 minutes until golden and risen.

Remove from the oven and allow them to cool in the tin for 5 minutes before lifting them out to fully cool on a wire rack.

Beat together the mascarpone and remaining lemon juice and, once the cupcakes have fully cooled, pipe or spoon some onto the tops.

Decorate with some freeze-dried fruit powder sprinkles or extra lemon zest, if you like.

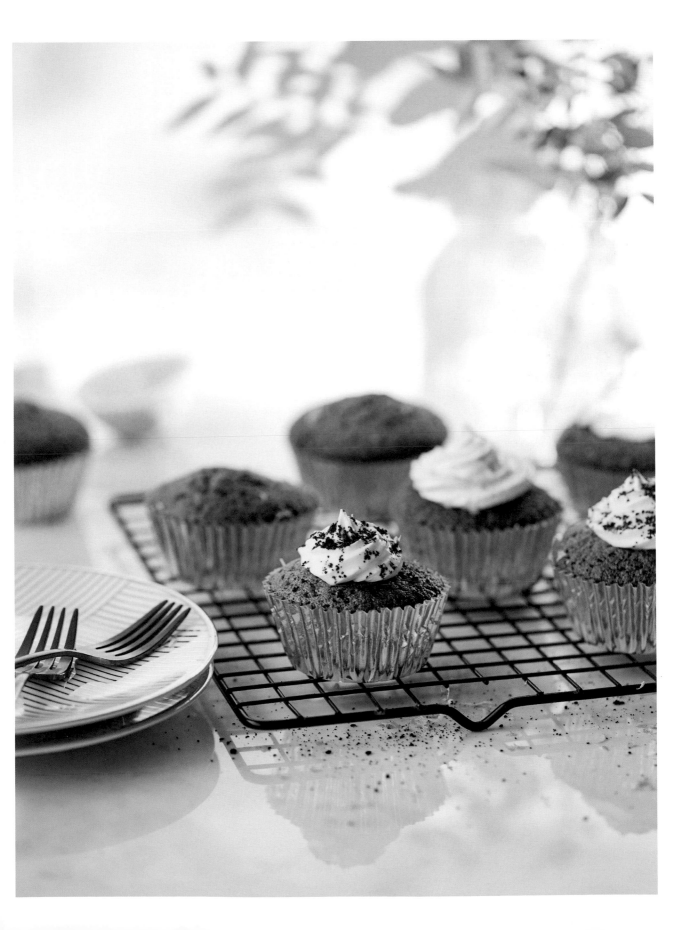

# carrot cake with cinnamon cream cheese topping

GOOD FOR
*entertaining*

I used to be terrible at making cakes, but I would INSIST on baking a cake for everybody's birthdays. The layers would be uneven, so it would look like the leaning tower of Pisa, and the icing would slide straight off the edge. I've given in and finally admit that when it comes to baking the quantities are important.

## makes 16 slices

200g spelt flour
80g caster sugar
2 tsp baking powder
1 tbsp ground cinnamon
2 tsp ground ginger
a pinch of salt
4 large eggs
80ml light olive oil
4 large carrots, grated (about 400g in total)
120g raisins

### for the icing
200g reduced-fat cream cheese
80g icing sugar
1 tsp ground cinnamon

### to decorate (*optional*)
40g chopped pistachios (or other chopped nuts)
toasted coconut slivers

Preheat your oven to 170°C/150°C fan/gas 3½. Line the base and sides of a 20cm springform cake tin with non-stick baking paper and use a little light olive oil to very lightly grease it.

Place the spelt flour, caster sugar, baking powder, spices and salt in a large mixing bowl and mix together.

Crack the eggs into a jug and add the olive oil. Beat together very well then pour the wet ingredients into the dry and use electric beaters to bring the mixture together.

Add the grated carrot and raisins and fold them in, using a large spoon.

Pour the mixture into the prepared tin and bake in the oven for around 45–50 minutes. It should be smelling delicious, risen and golden, and a cocktail stick inserted into the middle should come out clean. If not, pop it back in for another 5 minutes and then check again.

Once the cake is done, remove it from the oven and allow to cool in the tin for 15 minutes on a wire rack. Then carefully remove the springform tin and slide the cake off the base. Remove the paper from the edges and allow to cool to room temperature.

When the cake has cooled, put the cream cheese into a mixing bowl and use electric beaters to give it a whisk and loosen it. Then sift in the icing sugar and cinnamon and gently whisk it together.

Spread the icing over the top of the cake and create some beautiful waves in it. Use the pistachios or chopped nuts to decorate and scatter over some toasted coconut. It will look and taste amazing.

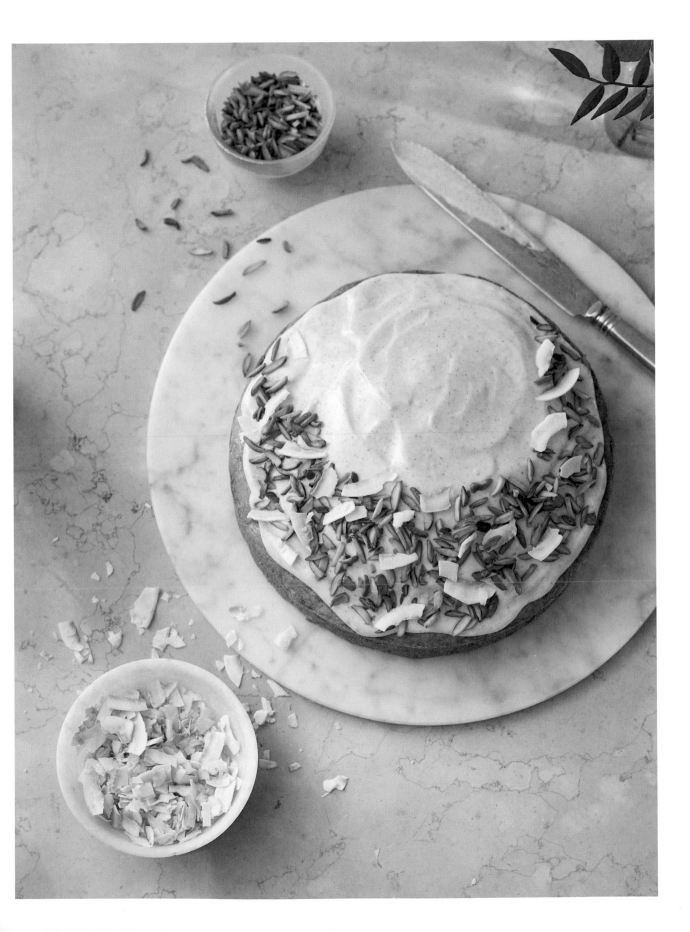

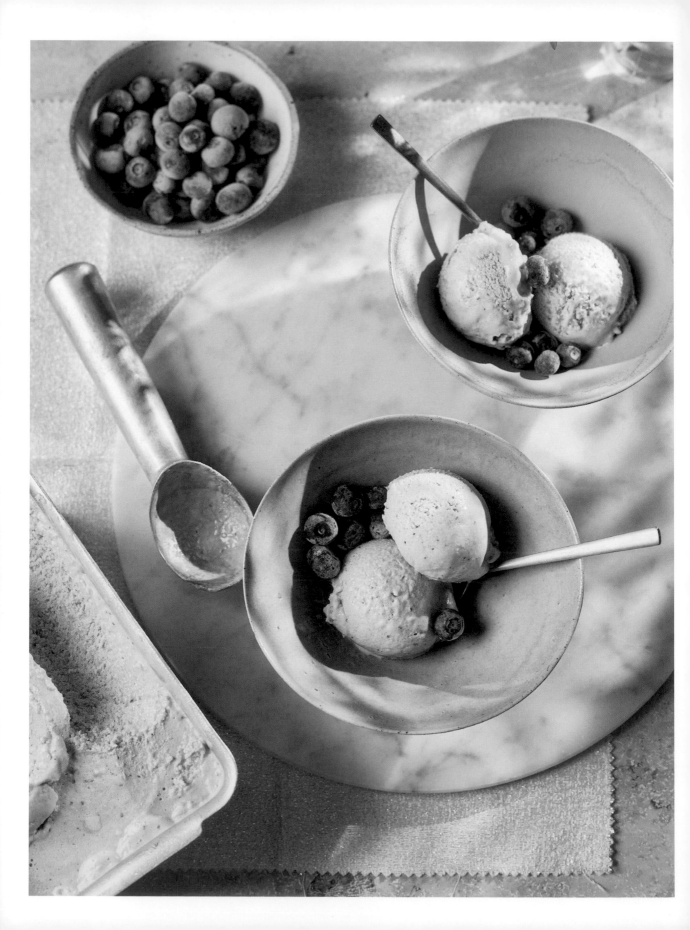

# blueberry protein ice cream

GOOD FOR
**post-workout**

Not only does this pudding look sensational but the flavour of the berries perfectly complements the creamy and sweet ice cream. I know the idea of using cottage cheese sounds weird but don't knock it before you try it! It is light and has the added benefit of extra protein too.

serves 8

400g cottage cheese
50g vanilla protein powder
250g blueberries, plus extra to serve
250ml almond milk
juice of 1 lemon

Place the cottage cheese, protein powder and blueberries in a food processor and blitz until smooth. This will take a good 3–4 minutes. Scrape the sides down occasionally to make sure you get everything.

Then, with the motor running, pour in the almond milk and lemon juice.

Sieve the mixture (to remove all the bits of skin that won't break down) straight into a 1-litre freezer container. Pop the container into the freezer for 2 hours, then remove and blitz again. Return the mixture to the rinsed-out container and put back in the freezer to set for around 4 hours (or overnight). Alternatively, churn in an ice-cream machine if you have one.

Before serving, remove from the freezer for 10–15 minutes to allow it to soften enough to scoop. Serve with extra blueberries.

> ⟨ TIP ⟩
> **Let this defrost a little at room temperature before serving**

# peach & basil 'sorbet'

Totally simple and absolutely sweet, what more could you want from a dessert? If you want a deliciously soft yet fruity pud then this is a good one for you. *(See pages 180–181 for photograph.)*

### serves 8

6 peaches, stoned and sliced

3 tbsp maple syrup

1 tbsp basil leaves

300ml full-fat coconut milk (you can use any leftovers in a smoothie!)

### to serve

thinly sliced fresh peaches

basil leaves

Place the peaches in a food processor and blitz until they have broken down into a purée. Add the maple syrup and basil leaves and blitz again until the basil leaves are incorporated into the peach purée. Scrape the sides down, put the lid back on and get the engine running. Slowly pour in the coconut milk until you have a very smooth purée.

Decant the mixture into a 1-litre freezer container. Pop it into the freezer for 2 hours, then remove and blitz again. Return to the rinsed-out container and put back in the freezer to set for around 4 hours (or overnight). Alternatively, churn in an ice-cream machine if you have one.

Before serving, remove from the freezer for 10–15 minutes to allow it to soften enough to scoop. Serve with some fresh peach slices and a couple of basil leaves.

> ⟨ TIP ⟩
> **Let this defrost a little at room temperature before serving**

# stewed forest fruits with a crunchy nutty topping

When I was at boarding school I would always look forward to lunch when it was fruit crumble. It was especially welcome after playing sport on a cold winter day. This is a lighter version of that stodgy pud. To mix it up, try combining different fruits. When I make my stewed fruits, I keep some to the side to add to breakfast the following morning – it is heavenly smothered over pancakes, plain yoghurt, cereal or even toast.

## serves 2

### for the berries
200g frozen mixed berries
1 tbsp lemon juice

### for the nutty topping
20g oats
15g flaked almonds, roughly chopped
15g pecans, roughly chopped
15g walnuts, roughly chopped
2 tbsp runny honey

Preheat your oven to 190°C/170°C fan/gas 5 and line a baking tin with non-stick baking paper.

Add all the ingredients for the nutty topping to a mixing bowl and stir to combine. Tip out into the baking tin and spread it out a little into an even layer. Place in the hot oven for 6 minutes, then remove the tin, stir and return for a further 6–7 minutes until everything is toasted.

While the topping is roasting, put the frozen berries and lemon juice into a saucepan. Place over a low heat and cook, stirring occasionally, for 10 minutes, until the berries have defrosted and broken down considerably, releasing all their lovely juices.

Divide the berries between two bowls and sprinkle over the nut topping. Serve immediately.

# lower-fat sticky toffee pudding

A lovely warming pudding made with sweet dates. I won a *Made in Chelsea, Come Dine With Me*-style charity dinner as a result of serving this showstopping pud to my fellow Chelsea companions! These tasty puddings are best served straight from the oven.

## serves 4

10g unsalted butter
180g dried dates, stones removed
175ml boiling water
200ml maple syrup
2 tsp vanilla extract
2 large eggs, separated
100g self-raising flour

**to serve**
1 vanilla pod or 1 tsp vanilla
　　bean paste
4 tbsp Greek yoghurt

Preheat your oven to 170°C/150°C fan/gas 3½ and lightly grease the insides of four ramekins with the butter.

Place the dates in a small saucepan and cover with the boiling water. Put over a medium heat and bring the water back up to the boil, then reduce the heat and simmer the dates for 5–6 minutes until they have softened and rehydrated.

Remove from the heat and drain the dates before putting them into a food processor along with half the maple syrup and the vanilla extract. Blitz until they are smooth. You may need to scrape the sides down a couple of times to help it.

Use a spatula to transfer the dates to a mixing bowl. Add the egg yolks to the dates and use an electric whisk to beat them in, then add the flour and beat it in quickly to mix.

Clean and dry your beaters well and then, in a separate mixing bowl, whisk the egg whites until they are at stiff peak stage. Fold them into the date mixture, using a large metal spoon and being careful not to squash out all the air.

Divide the remaining maple syrup between the four ramekins and then add the date mixture. Cover each one with some lightly greased foil and bake in the oven for 30–35 minutes.

If using a vanilla pod, cut in half and scrape out the seeds. Mix the seeds (or vanilla bean paste if using) into the Greek yoghurt and keep in the fridge until you are ready to serve.

Turn each pudding out onto a plate and top with a tablespoon of vanilla yoghurt.

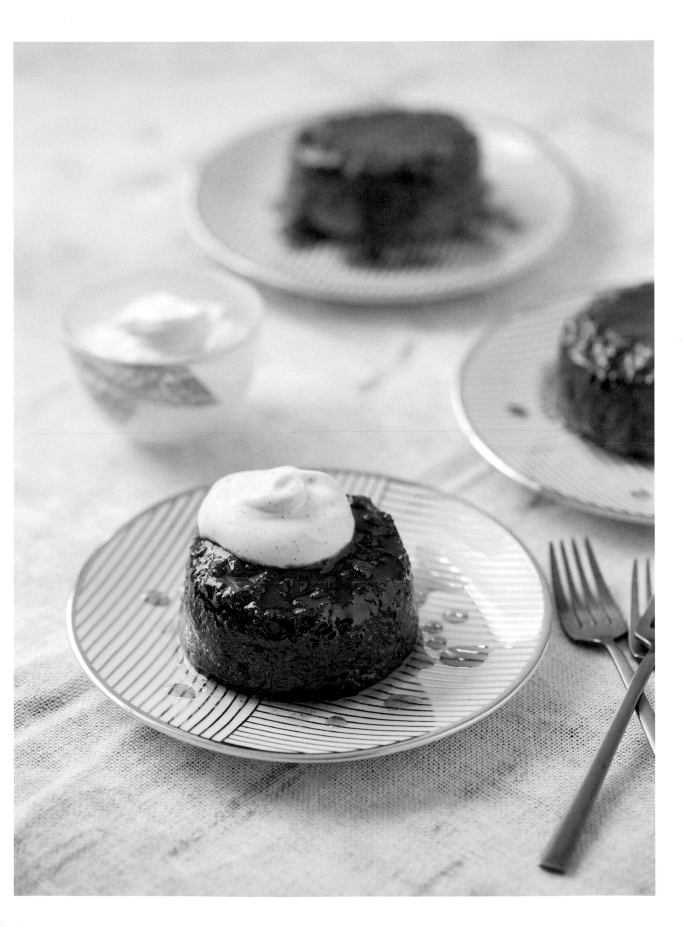

# banana & chocolate ice-cream sandwiches

This fun pudding is lip-smackingly good and great for all ages. It is also easy to assemble. I especially love making it with kids although every adult I know likes to behave like a child now and again too. The 'ice cream' is just banana mixed with cocoa powder and tastes amazing sandwiched between the golden crunchy spelt cookies.

## makes 10

### for the cookies

100g unsalted butter, softened

100g coconut sugar

1 large egg

225g spelt flour

50g dark chocolate (90% cocoa solids), melted

### for the banana chocolate ice cream

2 bananas, peeled, sliced and frozen

1 tbsp raw cacao powder

Put the butter and coconut sugar in a mixing bowl and, using electric beaters, beat together until pale and fluffy, then beat in the egg.

Add the flour and use a wooden spoon to incorporate it into the butter mixture. Once you have a cookie dough, bring it together with your hands. Divide it into two and roll into two sausage shapes. Wrap tightly in clingfilm and chill overnight in the fridge.

The next day, preheat your oven to 180°C/160°C fan/gas 4 and line two baking sheets with non-stick baking paper.

Cut the now firm dough into slices 6–7mm thick and lay them out on the baking sheets, spacing them apart a little. You should have enough to make 20 cookies. Pop the baking sheets into the hot oven and bake for 16–18 minutes until the edges are a lovely golden brown. Then remove and allow to cool to room temperature.

When the cookies have cooled, add the frozen banana slices and cocoa powder to a food processor and blitz until smooth. You'll need to coax it a little by scraping the sides down until it gets going, but it only takes a couple of minutes to have a lovely smooth ice cream.

Take a cookie and spread a layer of ice cream on one side. Sandwich the ice cream in place with another cookie. Repeat until you have made 10 ice-cream sandwiches.

Use a spoon to drizzle the melted chocolate decoratively over half of each cookie. Leave the chocolate to set. If you're not eating straight away, pop them into the freezer until you need them.

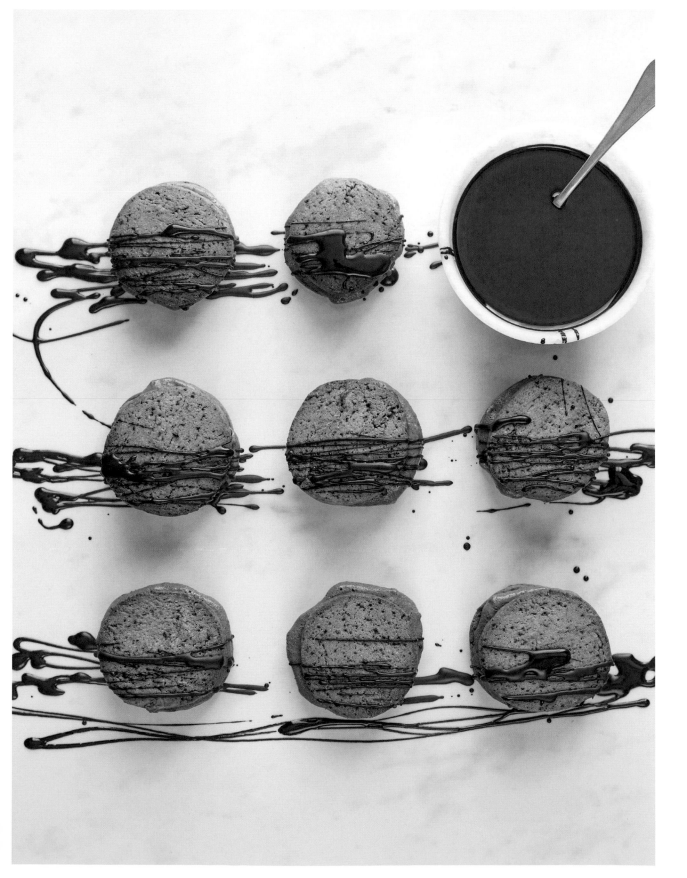

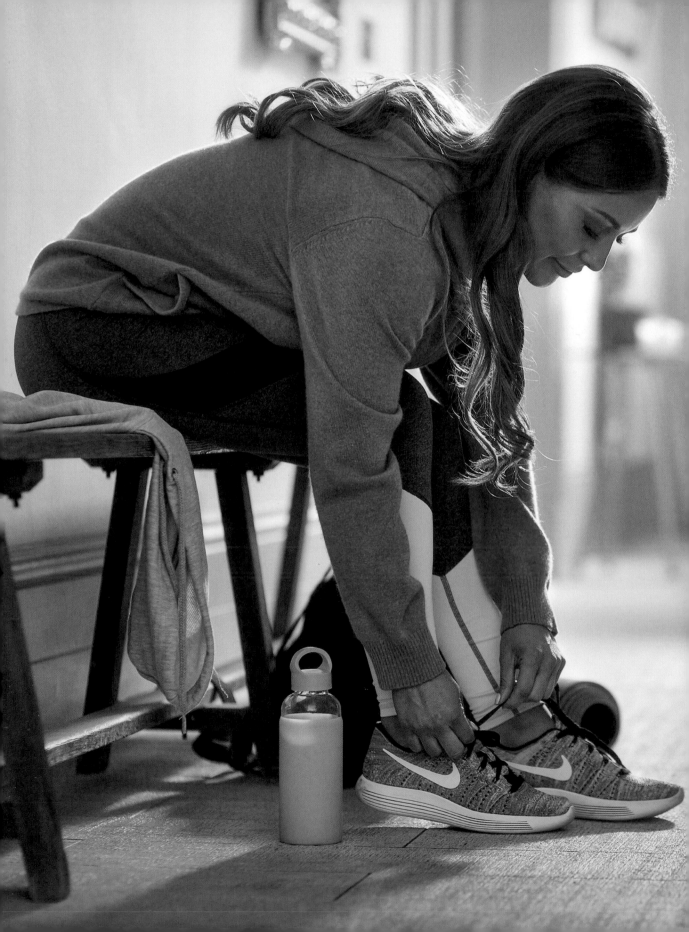

# the workouts

# PART 3

# Fitness is a lifetime commitment, not a sprint to the finish line. Do what makes you happy!

Many people are fearful of exercise because, like me, they have had bad experiences in the past. As I've discussed earlier, I used exercise as a form of punishment when going through a break-up, or in an attempt to drastically lose weight. I would run on a treadmill at the gym for as long as possible and follow a restricted calorie diet. With my body shape, short legs and a long-term problem with shin splints; the gym wasn't a place that put me at ease, especially when my confidence was at rock bottom. My attempts at extreme weight loss were pointless, because after a few sessions I would stop going, revert to my binge-eating cycle, go back to drinking and put it all back on again. It was only once I began to approach fitness as a long term commitment that my outlook started to change. First and foremost, I fell in love with how it made me feel, it was a total revelation that fitness could be fun!

A realistic relationship with fitness will help you stay on track! I aim to work out three times a week, although my job is sporadic so it has to fit around this. Having access to a fully decked out gym is great if that fits in with your lifestyle, but our body is the greatest machine we have and my workout plans are all designed so they can be done at home, with the most basic equipment. If you don't currently have access to the equipment at home already, you can buy it all relatively cheaply online or it should all be available in your local gym, if you are working out there.

Three workouts a week are enough for me to see and feel the benefits, but if you want to do them four or five times a week, I'm sure you'll feel amazing. The main goal is to find a balance between exercise, rest, and your other commitments. Personally, if I work out too often I find my body doesn't have a chance to properly recover, I end up feeling more worn-out and my results are actually diminished. If it is becoming too much, take a rest day!

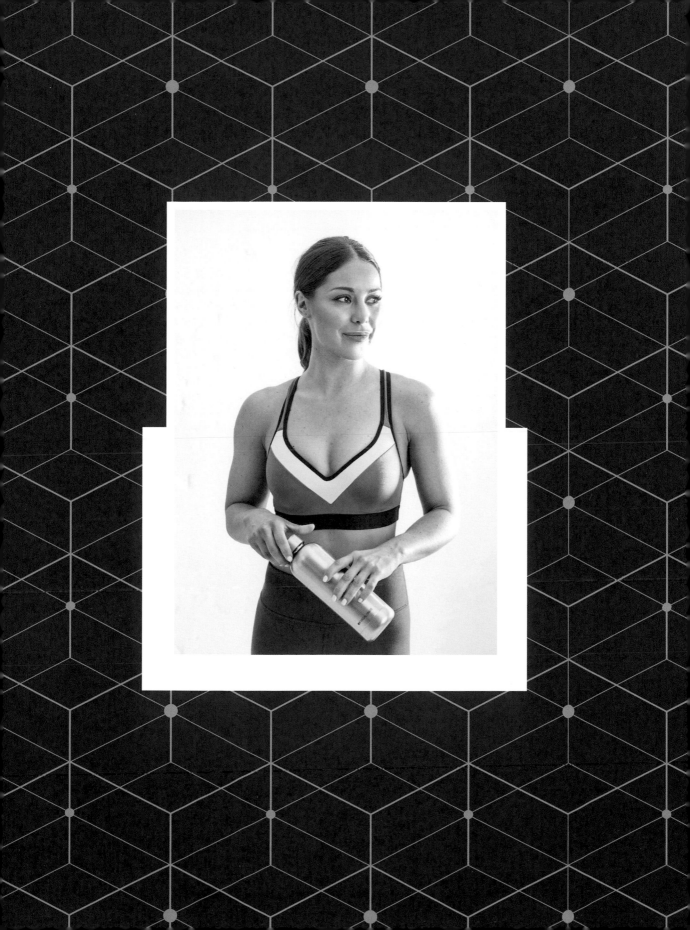

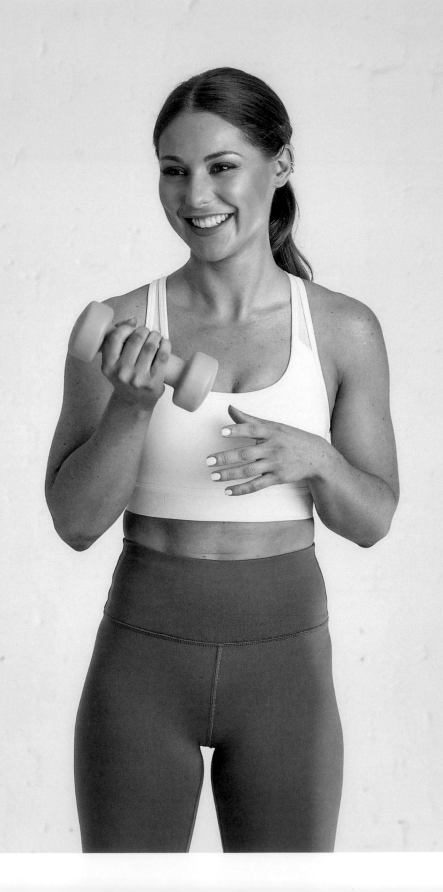

# adopt a more active lifestyle

While following my exercise plans, don't feel like you can't do other things; make the world your gym! Not only will variety help you stay motivated, there are always going to be times when it's harder to stick to your usual routine, or when it's more challenging to stay motivated – for example on holiday – find other activities you enjoy. I recently discovered a climbing wall around the corner from my house so I'm going to do a double-date wall climb... I'm sure it will provide a lot of laughs, but it's also a good way to increase agility and upper-body strength.

Being active doesn't equate to miserably running on a treadmill for an hour. Ryan and I love doing adult gymnastics, which I didn't even realise challenged my body until afterwards when I noticed I gained a lot of strength. We also go on long walks on the weekends or we cycle into different central London locations to browse shops and markets. Develop a fun relationship with exercise. Keep it fresh and it will never be a chore.

Try to be less lazy when it comes to every day activity. It may sound cringe, but I actually quite like doing chores, washing the dishes and carrying the shopping these days, because I know that I'm getting physically fitter, and then simple tasks become easier too. We take being on our feet for granted, but if you're moving about then you're burning energy (and can eat more as fuel as a result). You'll notice increased energy levels and your body will begin to adapt. Remember that every stretch, lunge, pace, jump up the stairs counts. I get laughed at a lot by Sam and Ryan for jump-squatting up the stairs, but I know they're jealous that I'm getting stronger! I love the saying 'first they laugh, then they follow' because there are a few instances in my life where this has proved to be true. Even my own brother used to mock me and Ryan for taking our exercise so seriously because he thought it was 'uncool', but now he has given it a chance he is totally addicted too.

The moment I stopped complaining about being active and on my feet, the happier I became. You know that feeling you get after a workout where you are inspired to be healthy and active for the rest of the day? The trick is to wake up every morning with that attitude and mentality and appreciate every move your body makes. I take the stairs instead of the lift and I don't rely on Ryan or other people to carry the shopping/luggage/anything else that I might have been lazy with in the past. When I'm on the way to filming somewhere local I will get a hire bike to avoid the traffic. If you work far from home and get the tube or bus then you could get off a stop early and walk the remaining distance to boost your step count. Or go for a quick walk around the block at lunchtime – it all adds up. It's important for my mental state to be out and about, interacting and connecting with people. I've recently noticed that my brother takes his calls out in the fresh air, he simply steps outside and walks as far as his legs will take him! I'm into it! Being active isn't about going from the sofa to having an explosive session in the gym, only to then return to the sofa, from one extreme to the other; it's about being springy in all aspects of life.

 **I remember popping to my mum's house around the corner and following her workout videos in the basement. I LOVED everything about it!**

## starting out

If you are a beginner, remember that some exercise is better than no exercise, and don't beat yourself up about it as you get used to being more active. Small steps will lead to big wins. It has taken two years for me to get to where I am today, and even I fluctuate from week to week. It is unrealistic to assume that you are going to be able to do the same amount of exercise every week without fail, as I have said before. I have no regular structure to my life most of the time, with filming *Made in Chelsea* and other jobs being the priority. My schedule is unpredictable. But I do the best with the time I have, making exercise and eating well fit around my day. Being able to work out at home is key to this. The majority of the exercises I do I can practise within a small space of roughly 2 square metres with a cheap gym mat and a couple of weights.

Strict targets are daunting and often you are setting yourself up for failure and then disappointment. I prefer balance to setting goals – but that's not to say targets don't ever work, especially if training for a specific event. If you are one of those people who needs targets in order to stay motivated, then start small so that you don't end up burning out – don't run before you can walk, as the saying goes. A realistic goal for someone starting out might be 'staying active for more than 15 minutes each day' – or to do one of my workouts three times a week.

# training at home

Before I formulated my own exercise routines I went to my mum's house around the corner and followed her workout videos in the basement. I LOVED everything about them! There are so many benefits to working out at home, including:

- You won't have to pay a monthly membership fee.
- You have the freedom and flexibility to exercise whenever.
- You don't have to spend time getting to and from the gym. TIME IS SO VALUABLE!
- You won't be distracted by prying eyes.
- You can prepare a healthy post-workout meal or have access to snacks.
- There's no complicated equipment to leave you feeling overwhelmed.
- You can wear whatever you want – I often wear pyjamas (and a good sports bra).
- You can play your music loud on a speaker without a care in the world.

## rest

If you push yourself hard during one workout session then you may need a couple of days to recover. I like to feel like I've used my muscles the day after a workout and then, particularly two days after a workout, when the DOMS (delayed onset muscle soreness) kicks in I know I've had an effective session. But you should never actually be in serious pain. I typically try to incorporate a reformer Pilates or yoga class once a week; a low-intensity class like this will help you to unwind, stretch and reset. One of the best classes I've ever done was one I accidentally agreed to attend with a friend. We turned up thinking we were doing a core workout in a studio, but the whole hour was dedicated to massaging all muscle groups with a small, hard ball. It was intense and a bit uncomfortable, but it targeted the tension I had built up during my workouts. Alternatively, you can check out some of my favourite cool-down stretches on page 248.

Other ways to speed up recovery and help muscle soreness includes drinking enough water, getting lots of good-quality sleep, eating plenty of lean protein and if you're feeling brave, having a cold bath or shower!

Ryan taught me to address muscle tightness using a foam roller to target certain areas before doing my warm-up or during my cool-down. I enjoy doing this because it increases blood flow and acts like a deep tissue massage which is super satisfying. Foam rolling should increase muscle pliability and help you move better, however, be careful if you're new to foam rolling because you don't want to overwork the muscle and damage the tissue, causing unnecessary pain. Try to remember to roll slowly and focus on positioning your body correctly. If in doubt, consult an experienced PT to help you.

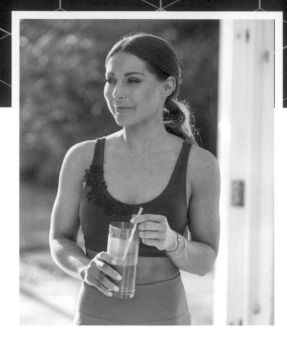

# top tips for staying motivated

1. Make your workouts fit your lifestyle – find and stick to the things that are working for you.

2. Take time before a workout to figure out what you are doing and don't rush the workout. I have created clear plans for you to make this preparation easier. (See pages 206–207.)

3. Breathe with purpose. I like to exhale loudly when I'm exerting pressure. If you blow out forcefully at the top of an ab exercise it makes them work harder.

4. Keep hydrated. Sip little and often during your workout and rehydrate afterwards.

5. Listen to your body: take rest days when you need them.

6. Keep a fitness journal and CELEBRATE SUCCESS.

7. Add in some new classes. Once the workout is booked then you will feel too guilty to bail. I never thought I would actually be saying this, but I look forward to waking up on a morning when I've booked a class.

8. If you use a gym rather than home to exercise, switch to a lunchtime workout in winter, when the dark evenings make it hard to find the motivation to go to the gym after work.

**Remember: you're only one workout away from a good mood. I never regret it when I do it, but I always regret it when I don't.**

# gaining strength

Whilst I am the biggest advocate of a slow-and-steady approach, there's no escaping that when it comes to doing the workouts it should be fairly intense, and you are likely to find some moves a bit hard. Make sure you do them with control and focus – if you don't give it your all and challenge your body, then you won't reap the rewards.

When I do my strength-building exercises (bodyweight exercises on the mat at home), I make sure I'm performing them at a moderate level so that I can maintain correct posture and balance, but I really push into the move so I can always feel the targeted muscles working. Flimsy movements aren't going to get you anywhere. For me, moderate intensity means having to breathe more quickly, but not being out of breath, developing a light sweat after around 10 minutes, but still being able to have some degree of conversation. When doing the cardio moves I always perform them with a vigorous intensity. This means my breathing is deep and fast, I typically sweat after 1 minute, and I can't speak without pausing for a breath. This level of exertion is what gets your heart rate up. It will also help you to burn calories, if that is your intention, and release endorphins which make you happy!

A combination of strength-building exercises and aerobic activity is what I've built my body on. In my opinion the most effective workouts combine both aspects if your goal is to live a healthier, fitter life. Previously I was too focused on cardio and ignored anything else. The strength training I've adopted increases the size and endurance of your muscles, which actually improves cardiovascular fitness. Having a better cardiovascular capacity increases the ability of the heart and lungs to supply oxygen-rich blood to the body's muscles, and then the muscles can better produce energy to move.

# let's get cracking

Ryan, who is a personal trainer, helped me create the workouts and exercises to ensure they are safe and correct. If in doubt, always seek advice from a qualified professional.

We wanted the workouts to be easy to understand without the added stress of getting to grips with a complicated programme. They combine a mix of exercises for arms and upper body, bum and legs, core, abs and high-intensity cardio, with a warm up and cool down. I have set these out in sections over the following pages, so that if you want to create your own workout or if you want to target just one body part at a time, then you can. These exercises can be done anywhere at any time, so no more excuses! Start today and you'll feel good for it.

# the fitness plans

## 5-min warm-up + 20-min workout (2 x 10-min rounds) + 5-min cool-down = 30-min (approx)

---

For optimum results I recommend that you do one of the workouts (A, B or C) twice a week, and the ab blast (D) on another day (please note the ab blast is 11 minutes long!).

### YOU WILL NEED:

✓ This book
✓ A timer
✓ A mat
✓ A water bottle
✓ A skipping rope
✓ Dumbbells (2-5kg, depending on ability)
✓ A small, light-looped resistance band
✓ Music!

### TIPS TO TACKLE YOUR WORKOUT:

• Choose which level workout you want to do and lay out all your equipment.
• Get to know the exercises before you start to make your workout easier.
• Set your timer to keep track (I use my phone). Although I appreciate that everyone moves at a different pace, I'd suggest a rest period of 10 seconds maximum between each move. Aim to complete each round for A, B or C in 10 minutes and complete 2, with a 60 second break after the first.

## a word on weights:

If you are a beginner I would start with 2-2.5kg dumbbells for the bicep curl, shoulder press and lateral raise – that is what I used when I began my fitness journey. Starting small is more manageable, you can work your way up to heavier weights as you gain strength and the exercises start becoming easier. There will always be benefits of doing high repetitions of small weights as long as you keep engaging your muscles. I find that the lateral raise is harder than the other two arm exercises, so don't be embarrassed to begin with an even smaller weight, prioritising form over anything else! When I'm using a weight as part of a core exercise, e.g. the Russian twist, I aim for 5kg which comes in whatever form is available (a dumbbell, weighted ball or plate usually).

# If I'm in the gym, I warm up on the treadmill for 5 minutes – running at a moderate speed with 2 x 30-second sprints, at 2 minutes and then at 4 minutes to get my heart rate up.

It's really important to warm up before exercising so that you get the most out of a workout, an effective warm-up will get your heart rate up, activate your muscles and get them ready for activity. If you don't warm up you are exposing yourself to a risk of injury so it is worth investing a little extra time. I've shared an example of a 5-minute warm-up to work the full body using controlled movements to ensure your muscles are switched on. It is called a WARM up for a reason - you want to get warmth into your body and muscles in order to improve their function and range of motion.

Ideally you would complete the warm-up exercises without breaks; however, as long as you get the blood flowing to your muscles that is the main goal. DO YOUR BEST. If you are working out more than a couple of times a week and you are experiencing particularly sore muscles I would recommend spending longer on your warm-up period. Aim for 10 minutes, so double up the routine.

## warm up
### SET TIMER: 5 MINUTES

| | |
|---|---|
| **SKIPPING** | **x 60 seconds (page 240)** |
| 5 seconds rest | |
| **HIGH-KNEE RUNNING** | **x 30 seconds (page 242)** |
| 5 seconds rest | |
| **MOUNTAIN CLIMBERS** | **x 30 seconds (page 243)** |
| 5 seconds rest | |
| **HEEL FLICKS** | **x 30 seconds (page 244)** |
| 5 seconds rest | |
| **BURPEES** | **x 30 seconds (page 245)** |
| 5 seconds rest | |
| **TUCK JUMPS** | **x 30 seconds (page 246)** |
| 5 seconds rest | |
| **JUMPING JACKS** | **x 60 seconds (page 247)** |

## beginner (A)

WARM UP: 5 minutes (page 205)
SET TIMER: 10 minutes

1. **HIGH PLANK**
   x 30 second hold (pages 244-5)
2. **FLUTTER KICKS**
   x 20 reps (page 230)
3. **SIDE PLANK**
   x 20 second hold per side (page 226)
4. **BIRD DOG**
   x 20 reps, 10 each side (page 228)
5. **TOE TAPS**
   x 20 reps, 10 each side (page 236)
6. **HEEL TOUCH**
   x 20 reps, alternating sides (page 237)
7. **STRAIGHT LEG RAISE**
   x 12 reps (page 229)
8. **GLUTE BRIDGE**
   x 20 reps (page 220-221)
9. **BODYWEIGHT SQUAT**
   x 20 reps (page 216-17)
10. **HEEL FLICKS**
    x 20 seconds (page 224)
11. **JUMPING JACKS**
    x 20 seconds (page 247)
12. **BICEP CURL**
    x 12 reps per arm (page 208-9)
13. **SHOULDER PRESS**
    x 12 reps (page 212)
14. **TRICEP DIPS**
    x 12 reps (page 210-11)

REST FOR 60 SECONDS AND REPEAT

COOL DOWN: 5 minutes (page 248)

## intermediate (B)

WARM UP: 5 minutes (page 205)
SET TIMER: 10 minutes

1. **JUMP SQUAT**
   x 20 reps (page 218-19)
2. **MOUNTAIN CLIMBERS**
   x 20 reps (page 243)
3. **GLUTE KICKBACKS**
   x 30 reps, 15 each side (page 222-23)
4. **ELBOW TO PLANK PUSH-UP**
   x 15 reps (page215)
5. **SIDE PLANK WITH OBLIQUE DIP**
   x 15 reps per side (page 226)
6. **SCISSOR KICKS**
   x 20 reps over and under, 40 in total (page 230)
7. **HIGH PLANK**
   x 30 second hold (page 224-5)
8. **HIGH-KNEE RUNNING**
   x 30 seconds (page 242)
9. **LATERAL RAISE**
   x 15 reps each arm (page 213)
10. **TRICEP DIPS**
    x 15 reps (page 210-11)
11. **JACKKNIFE**
    x 15 reps (page 239)
12. **RUSSIAN TWIST**
    x 20 reps on each side (with or without weight) (page 234)
13. **WEIGHTED CRUNCH**
    x 20 reps (page 233)
14. **PLANK WITH SHOULDER TAP**
    x 20 reps, 10 on each side (page 224-5)

REST FOR 60 SECONDS AND REPEAT
COOL DOWN: 5 minutes (page 248 )

## hard (C)

WARM UP: 5 minutes (page 205)
SET TIMER: 10 minutes

1. **CRAB WALK WITH RESISTANCE BAND**
   x 60 seconds, 30 seconds each side (page 220-1)
2. **TUCK JUMPS**
   x 20 reps (page 246)
3. **SEATED SCISSOR CROSS**
   x 20 reps over and under, 40 in total (page 238)
4. **SIDE PLANK WITH OBLIQUE DIP**
   x 20 reps each side (page 226)
5. **PUSH-UP**
   x 20 reps (page 214)
6. **WEIGHTED CRUNCH**
   x 20 reps (page 233)
7. **BICYCLE CRUNCH**
   x 20 reps each side (page 235)
8. **GLUTE BRIDGE**
   x 20 reps (hold at top for 20 seconds on final rep) (page 220-1)
9. **BURPEES**
   x 30 seconds (page 245)
10. **SKIPPING**
    x 60 seconds (page 240-1)
11. **V-SIT**
    x 20 reps (page 227)
12. **JACKKNIFE**
    x 15 reps (page 239)
13. **RUSSIAN TWIST WITH WEIGHT**
    x 20 reps each side (page 234)
14. **JUMP SQUATS**
    x 30 seconds (page 218-19)

REST FOR 60 SECONDS AND REPEAT
COOL DOWN: 5 minutes (page 248)

## 11-min ab blast (D)

With the ab blast routine do 30 seconds of exercise, followed by 15 seconds of rest, working your way through the list as best you can - then repeat.

WARM UP: 5 minutes (page 205)
SET TIMER: 11 minutes

1. **JACKKNIFE**
   (page 239)
2. **CRUNCHY FROG**
   (page 231)
3. **TOE TAPS**
   (page 236)
4. **FLUTTER KICKS**
   (page 230)
5. **PLANK WITH SHOULDER TAP**
   (page 224-5)
6. **CRUNCH**
   (page 232)
7. **STRAIGHT LEG RAISE**
   (page 229)
8. **BIRD DOG**
   (page 228)
9. **SIDE PLANK WITH OBLIQUE DIP** (15 seconds each side)
   (page 226)
10. **RUSSIAN TWIST**
    (page 234)
11. **V-SIT**
    (page 227)
12. **HEEL TOUCH**
    (page 237)
13. **BICYCLE CRUNCH**
    (page 235)
14. **SCISSOR KICKS**
    (page 230)
15. **HIGH PLANK**
    (page 224-5)

REST FOR 60 SECONDS AND REPEAT
COOL DOWN: 5 minutes (page 248)

# arms & upper body

## bicep curl

This exercise targets the muscle on the front of your upper arm. It is an isolation workout, but useful because your biceps are involved in numerous everyday activities.

You can either do this one arm at a time using 1 dumbbell whilst your other hand rests on your waist for stability, or you can alternate between both arms using 2 dumbbells. If you're using 2 dumbbells then use the weight of the resting dumbbell to balance you.

### FOR A SINGLE ARM BICEP CURL:

- Stand up straight with a dumbbell in one of your hands and let your other arm fully extend to the ground. Keep your elbow tucked into your torso. Rotate your hand so that your palm is facing up towards the ceiling. This is your starting position. Then exhale and curl the weight up until you feel the bicep muscle contract and your dumbell is at shoulder level, keeping your upper arm stationary. Release back to the starting position. It is important to move slowly on your way down to put pressure on the muscle.

- Don't use momentum to swing the weight up, as the exercise won't be as effective.

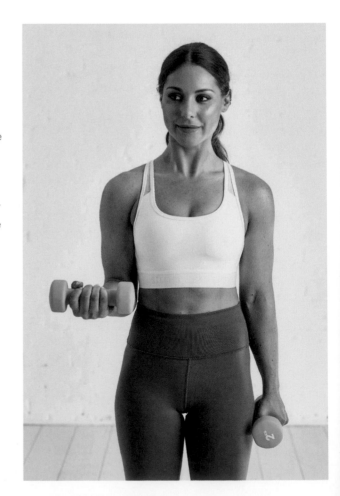

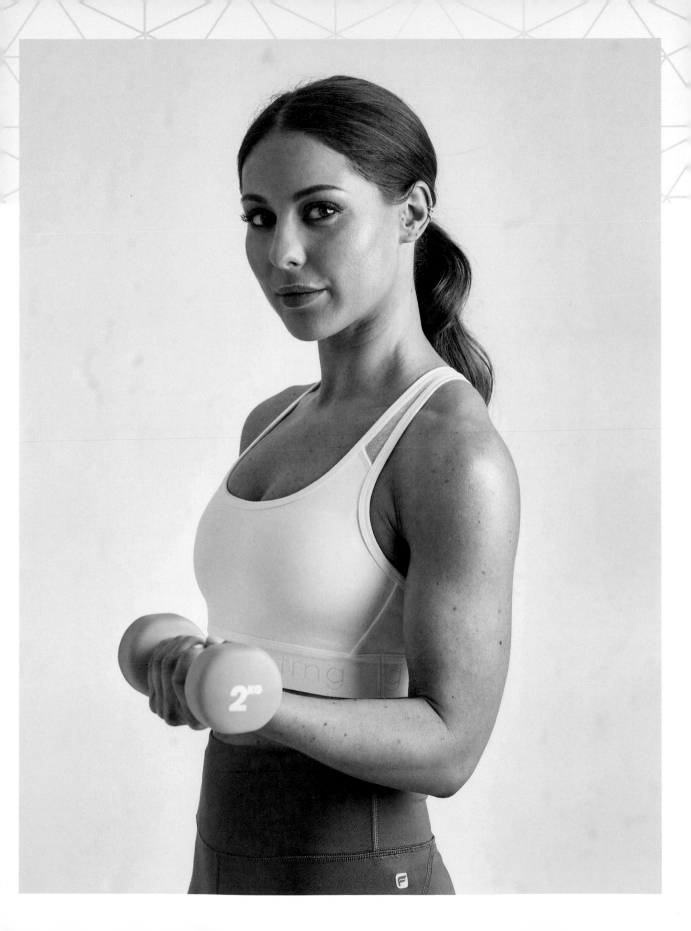

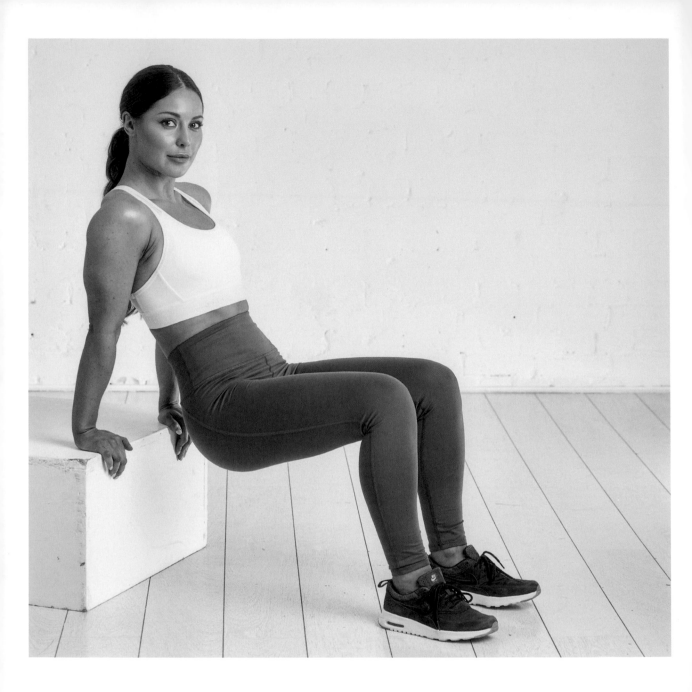

# tricep dip

Using a bench, sofa or any other raised stable surface, sit facing away from the surface. (From experience I would advise steering clear of a chair on wheels, LOL).

With a tricep dip you can either have your legs straight or bent – it doesn't matter, but practise whichever feels the most comfortable for you with whatever surface you have chosen to use. I personally think it is easier to have your knees bent, so maybe start with that variation and then progress to straight legs out in front of you.

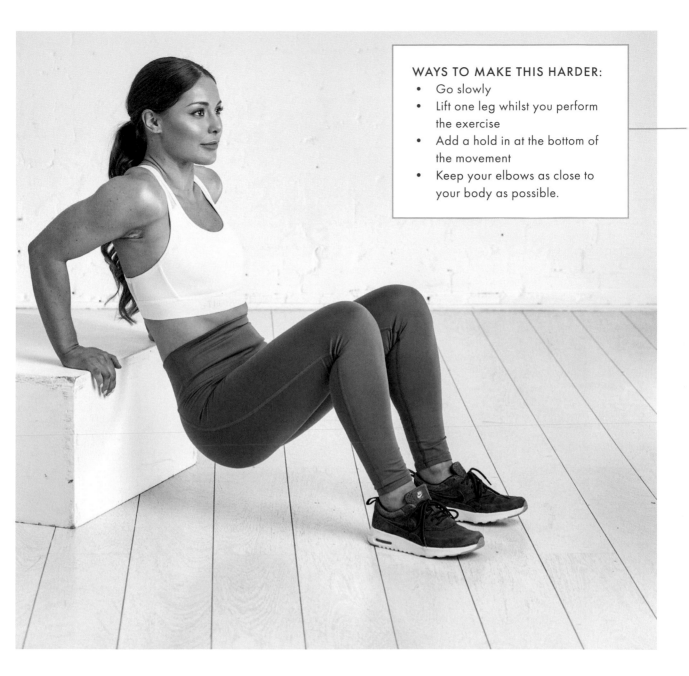

- Place your hands behind your back on the edge of the surface, shoulder width apart, knuckles facing forwards. Legs should be out in front, either bent or fully extended.

- Hold your body up by extending the elbow joints so your arms are fully extended. This is your starting position.

- Next, bend and lower the elbows and dip down to a 90-degree angle, using your tricep muscles to allow this movement. You should dip down as low as you can before powering up through the triceps, extending the arms and straightening the bend in the elbow.

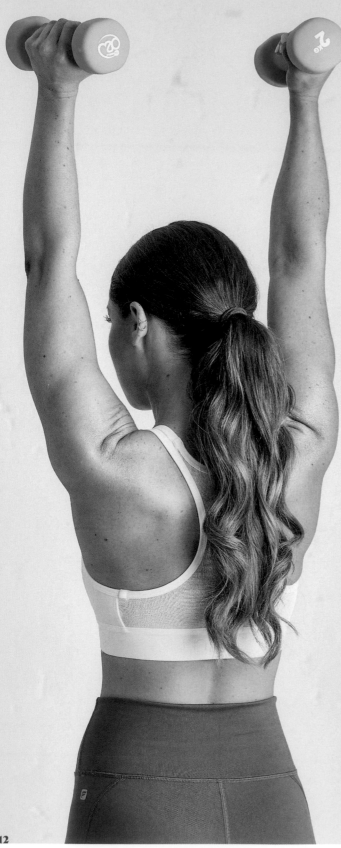

## shoulder press

This exercise is good for working the shoulder muscles. You can do this exercise standing or seated. If you are going to use a heavy weight I would recommend sitting down so that you have maximum support from your lower body.

- Hold 2 dumbbells, one in each hand, at shoulder height with bent arms, either side of your head (not resting on your body) with your palms facing inwards. This is your starting position.

- Exhale and push the dumbbell in an upward motion so that your arms are straight above your head. Then after a pause at the top, bring the dumbbells back to the starting position whilst inhaling.

- Make sure you don't rush this movement. Slow and steady wins this race.

# lateral raise

Don't be fooled by how simple it looks, this one is deceptively hard. Pick a light weight, as even then it is very challenging. You want to be able to complete the exercise without compromising good form.

- Similar to the bicep curl, you can either use 1 dumbbell and do one arm at a time or hold 2 dumbbells and alternate between arms. If you are using 1 dumbbell then you can place your hand on your hip for stability. If using 2 dumbbells, then stand with a dumbbell in each hand at either side of your body.

- Stand with feet hip width apart. Keep your back straight with your core activated and your bum tucked in. Then slowly lift the weights out to the side until your arms are parallel to the floor. Hold for a second, then lower your arms to the starting position. The slower you move the dumbbells down the harder your shoulders will work to manage the weight.

- Make sure that your arms don't go too high – avoid reaching above the parallel point.

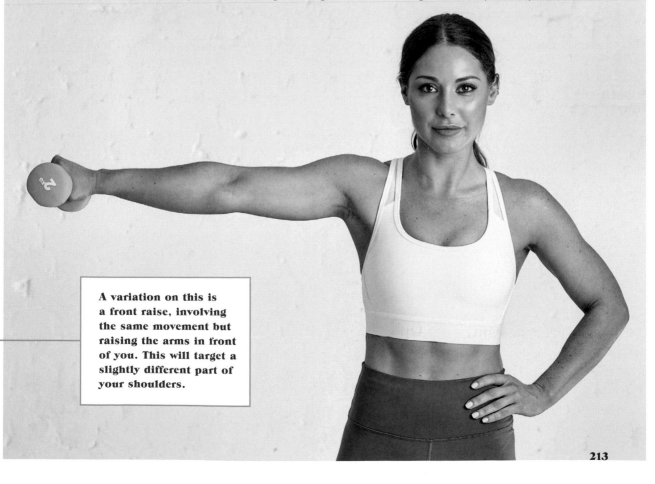

A variation on this is a front raise, involving the same movement but raising the arms in front of you. This will target a slightly different part of your shoulders.

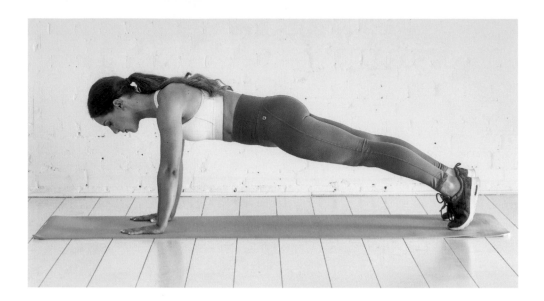

# push-up

A push-up is a full body functional movement and a good measure of one's core strength. It can be challenging, particularly to those who don't often exercise their arms, chest and shoulders, but is a solid indicator of progress. If you're starting out, go slowly and focus on technique. If you're not doing it right, you risk straining your lower back.

- Position yourself face down with your hands underneath your shoulders on the floor and your legs extended back shoulder width apart, balanced on your toes. Your back should form a straight line to your feet, descending downwards towards the floor. Keep your spine neutral, tuck your bum in, and engage your core.

- Bend your arms at the elbow joint (roughly 90 degrees) whilst lowering your torso down towards the floor. Make sure your chest doesn't collapse onto the floor. Hover in this position for a split second, making sure your form is correct before pressing back up to the start position using your chest and triceps.

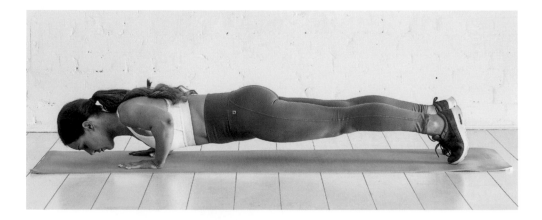

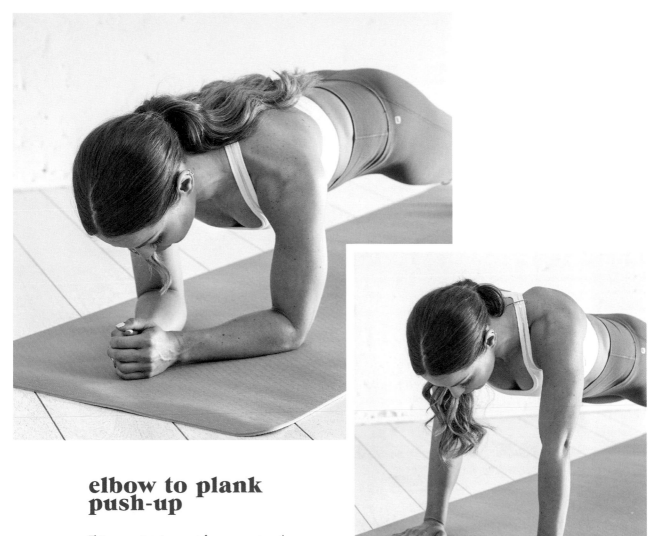

# elbow to plank push-up

This exercise is great for engaging the core and abdominals as well as the shoulders and arms.

- Start in a low plank position on your forearms, with your elbows and feet shoulder width apart. Your back should be as flat as possible.

- Using one arm at a time, press your body up into a push-up position (see top pic on page opposite, the high plank). In order to do this most effectively, try to keep your whole body still (with the exception of your arms). This is achievable by contracting (tensing) other muscles in your body, such as your glutes.

- Then lower yourself back down one arm at a time, in the same order, into the low plank.

- To make it harder, add a push-up between the push-up position and returning to the low plank position.

# bum & legs

## bodyweight squat

I have noticed a great improvement in the firmness of my bum and thighs since learning how to do squats properly. This is a compound movement that helps get your glutes, quads, hips, hamstrings, calves and core into gear. It should be a staple part of your routine because not only does it help with strength but it also aids flexibility and balance.

- Stand with your feet shoulder width apart with your chest up and your arms extended out in front parallel to the floor for balance. This is your starting position.

- Begin the movement by bending your knees and pushing your hips back as if you are sitting onto a chair. Continue down as low as you can while keeping your spine neutral and making sure your knees don't creep over your toes. Keep your head and chest up and facing forwards.

- Then reverse the motion and push back up through the heels to return to a standing position, while tensing your glutes as much as possible.

- If you feel your back taking control at any point, make an active effort to engage the glutes and you will notice a big change.

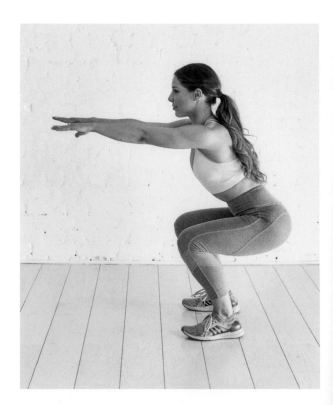

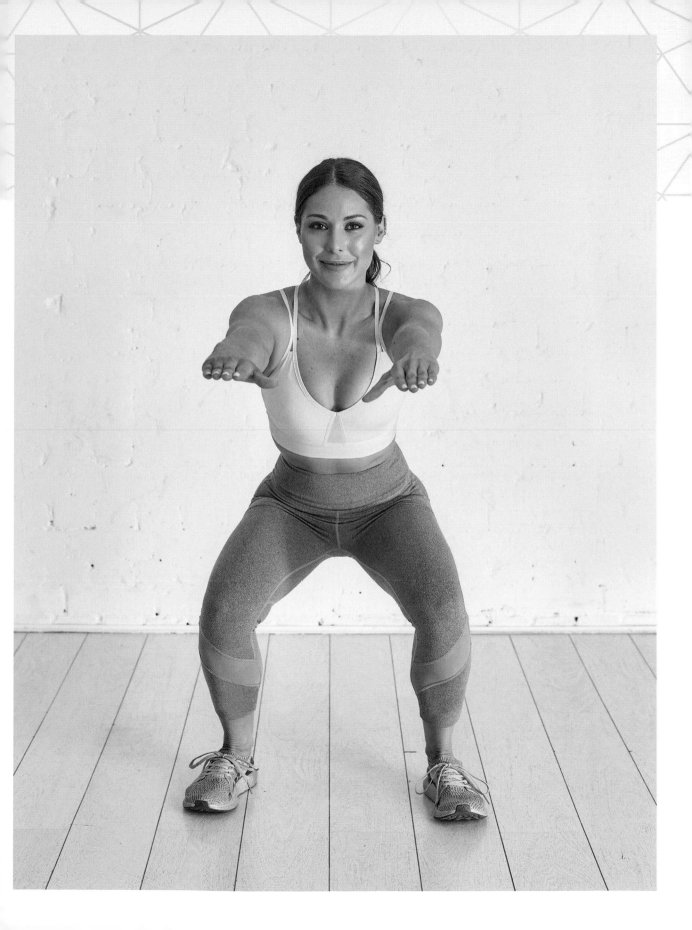

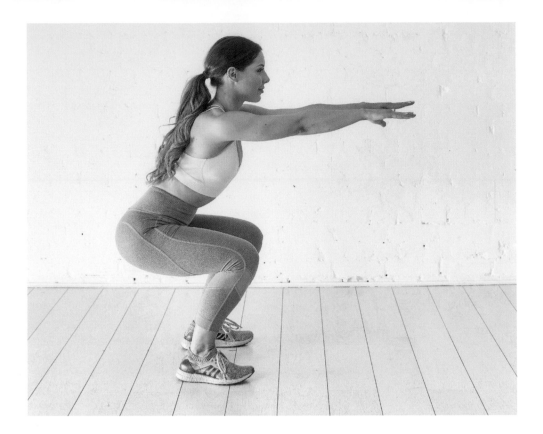

# jump squat

A jump squat is the same as a bodyweight squat, except this time you are aiming to make the upward phase of the movement explosive – as hard and fast as you can – generating an upward lift and carrying you into a vertical jump. Because jump squats are hard, they need to be performed properly in order to prevent injury.

- Start in a standing position, with your feet directly underneath your shoulders and your toes turned slightly outwards. I find turning my toes out ensures that my knees don't bend in, thus alleviating pressure on them. Lower yourself into a squat as described on page 216, with your arms either down at your sides or held out together in front of you to assist in balancing at the low point of the squat.

- Breathe out and jump as high as you can in a controlled manner, driving hard with your legs to extend them straight underneath you. Throw your arms behind you to accelerate the movement.

- When you land, try to lower your body back into a balanced squat position, as softly as possible. This requires control and makes it hard. Try to perfect one jump squat before performing several in sequence.

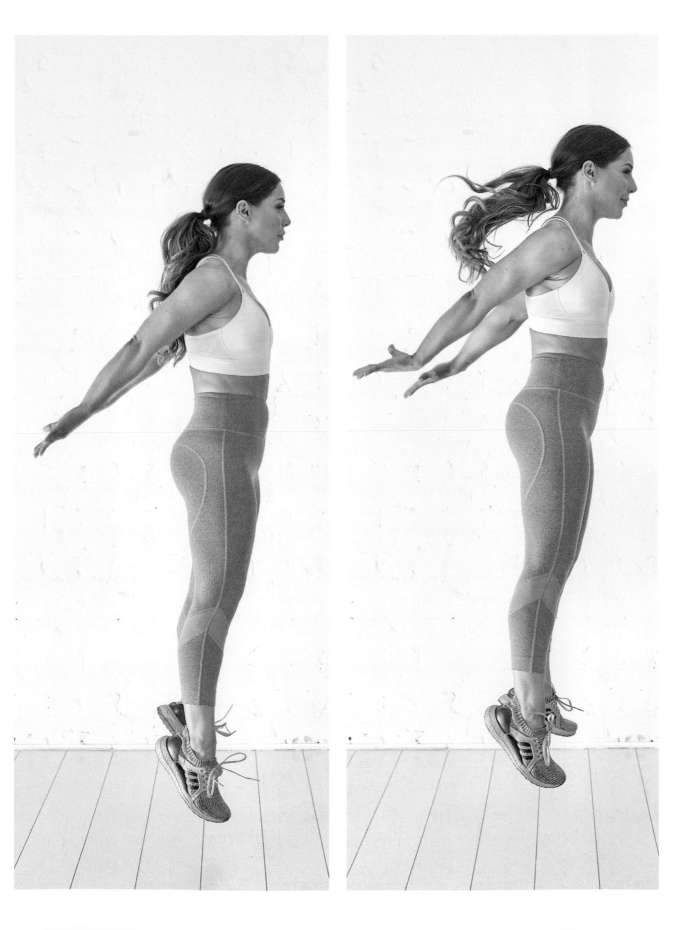

# crab walk with resistance band

The crab walk is a good way to strengthen the glutes in a slow and controlled manner. You can build up strength and change the tension in the resistance band as you get stronger over time, which is pretty satisfying.

- Place a resistance band around your calves so that it is has enough tension to stay up. Open the legs to wider than hip width with your toes slightly turned out. Rotate your knees out so that they are above your slightly turned-out feet. You should feel a contraction in your glute muscles. You can adopt a prayer pose for balance (see pic on right).

- Lower yourself into a half squat position with knees slightly bent, creating tension on the band. Take a step sideways, pushing out against the band, then bring the other leg a step inwards, keeping resistance in the band. Repeat with the other leg, and repeat this series of side steps, making sure your inner foot doesn't spring back in.

# glute bridge

I like using this exercise as a glute warm-up because it is relatively easy. It is great for improving hip mobility and strengthening the lower back.

- Lie on your back with your knees together and bent, and your feet flat on the floor, hip distance apart. Keep your arms either side of your body, palms down. Then drive your weight through your heels, raising your hips upwards off the ground. Squeeze your glutes and keep your abdominals tensing so you don't extend your back. Hold the position at the top for a couple of seconds and lower back down slowly, but before your hips touch the floor and the contractions switch off, drive back up.

- To make it harder you can add a resistance band just above the knees and push out to create tension (see pic on bottom right).

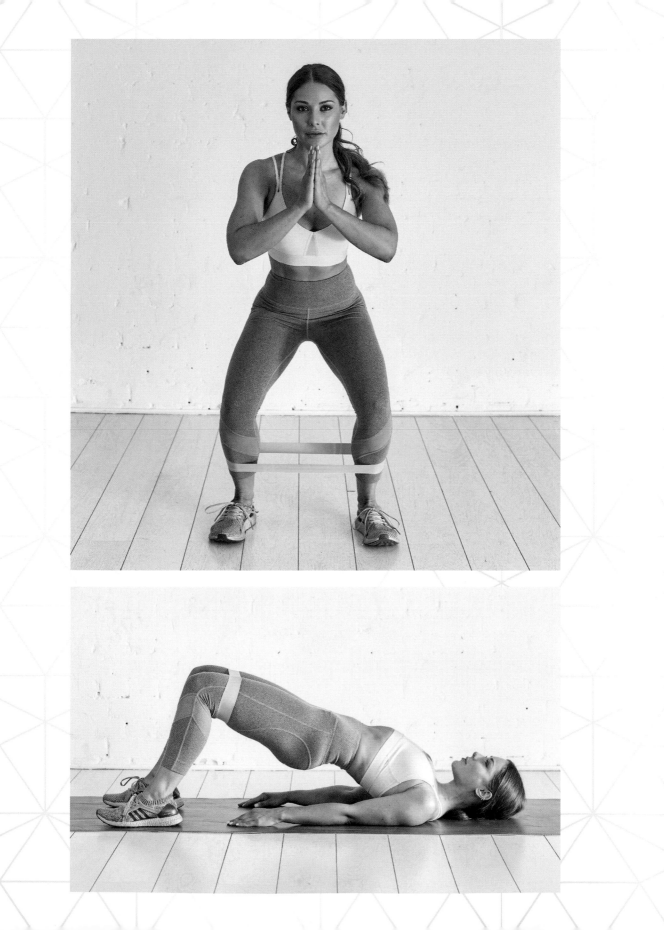

# glute kickback

This is one of my favourite lazy moves. It targets your gluteus minimus (the part where your glute meets your hamstring). Simply put, it will give you a full and round bum if you practise regularly enough.

- Start on all fours with your knees and hands on the floor roughly hip distance apart. Exhale and push one foot back behind you, bending your leg at about a 90 degree angle towards the ceiling. Contract the glutes of the leg that you are pushing behind you whilst lifting it in the air. At the top of this move the quad should be parallel to the floor whilst the calf should be perpendicular. Return to the starting position and repeat.

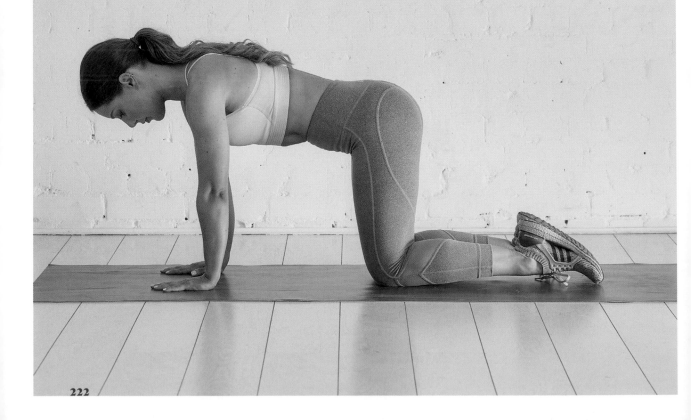

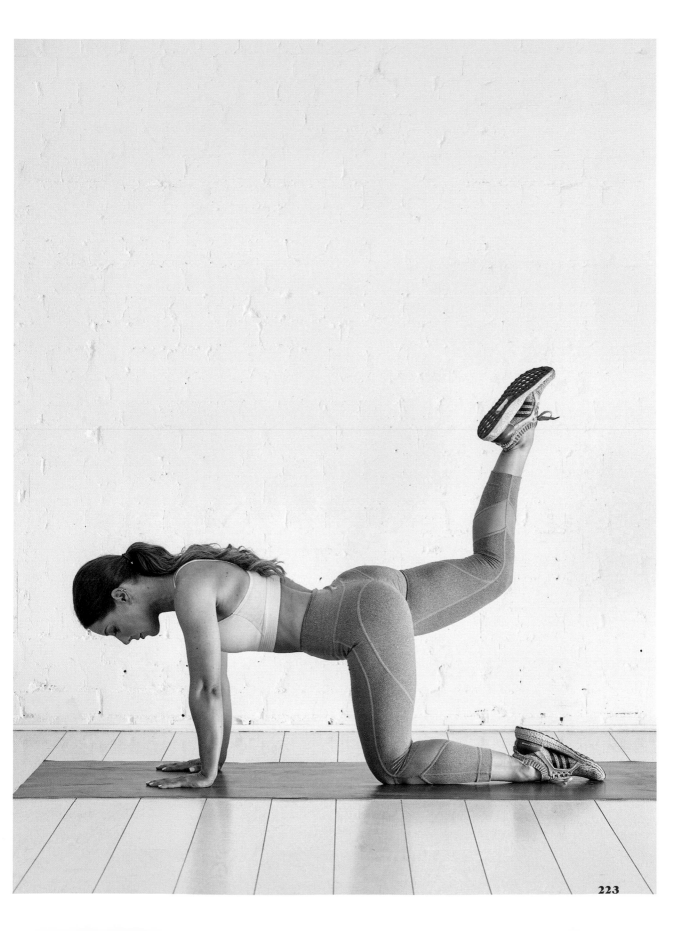

# core

## high plank

Everyone should learn how to do a plank because it builds strength and endurance in your core. When it comes to planking, form is everything, otherwise you won't use the right muscles! I find that the more I plank, the more conditioned my body becomes, so I can hold it for much longer with ease. Here I demonstrate a high plank which is a good variation to start with.

• Start on all fours in a table top position, kneeling on the floor. Your hands should be shoulder width apart pressed flat against the floor directly under your shoulders with your arms fully extended. When you feel balanced, lift your body off of the floor with your legs extended back so that you are supporting your weight between your hands and your toes. Hold the elevated position off the floor by squeezing your core abdominal muscles tight and keeping your back straight. Make sure you don't allow your shoulders or back to sag towards the ground; continue to breathe regularly through the exercise.

**FOR THE PLANK WITH SHOULDER TAP VARIATION:**

• You do the plank with fully extended arms in the high plank position (see top pic on opposite page). It is important to have a stable base so that you don't put too much strain on your shoulders. Engage your abs and your glutes, and then, keeping the rest of your body as still as possible, tap your right hand to your left shoulder before replacing it to the ground. Alternate by tapping your other hand to the opposite shoulder. Keep your hips square to the ground.

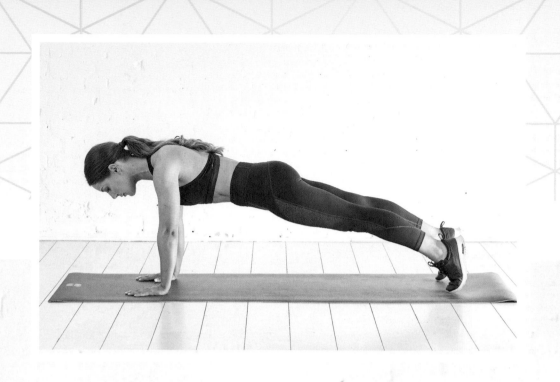

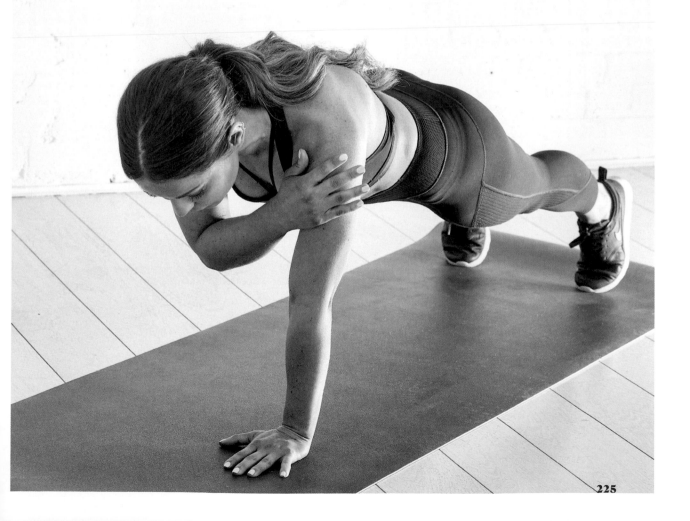

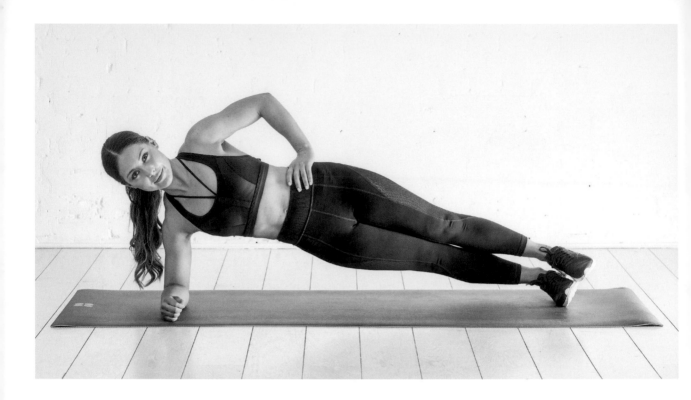

# side plank

People often neglect the side plank in favour of the regular front plank but it's important to note that they work different parts of your core. This move is good at strengthening your mid section, including your obliques. This can help prevent back problems as you get older, and keeps the spine better protected.

- Lie on your side, with your elbow under your shoulder and your forearm flat on the floor at 90 degrees to your body. Your feet should be together, resting one on top of the other.

- Elevate the weight of your body off the floor by raising your hips, allowing the side of your foot and forearm to hold the weight up. Your body should be in a straight line from head to feet. Hold the position without allowing your hips to drop. If you engage your abdominals correctly then your body should remain rigid and won't sway. Repeat on the other side according to workout.

## side plank with oblique dip

Same as for the side plank, but rather than holding the elevated position off the floor, allow the mid section of your body to drop down slowly, then contract the muscles to pop the hips back up to the start position. Repeat at your own pace, then switch sides.

# v-sit

The v-sit is actually quite an advanced exercise that tests your balance and core. Remember to breathe!

- Start in a seated position with your legs bent and feet raised off the floor. Hold your arms out straight, parallel to the floor in front of you. Rock back until you're balanced comfortably and your legs and back are at a 45 degree angle to the ground. Your body should create 2 v-shapes, one facing up, one facing down.

- Stretch your legs out and lower your feet towards the floor, doing the same with your head and shoulders the other way. Hold the position then pull back up to your starting position, contracting your abdominals.

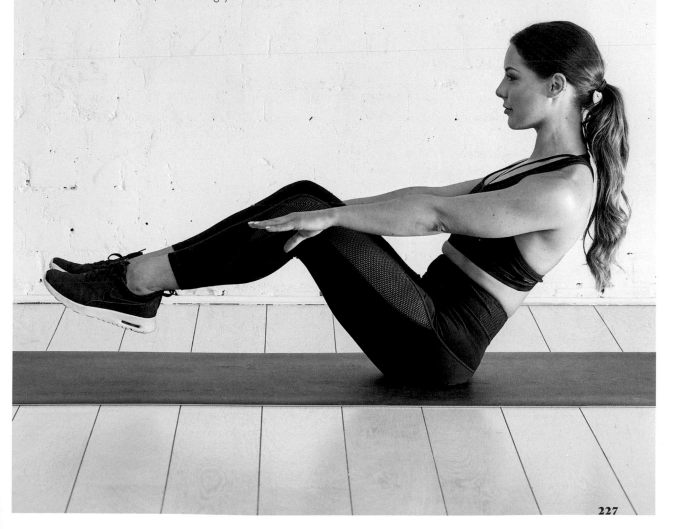

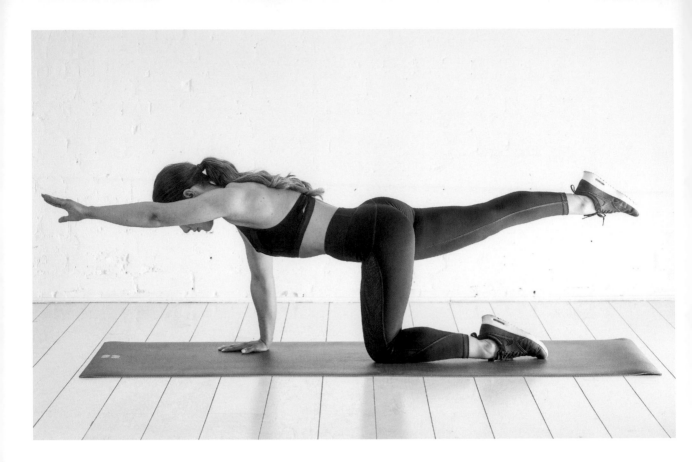

# bird dog

This exercise is great for training the body to stabilise your lower back. It requires no equipment and works the abs, back and bum.

- Start in a kneeling position on all fours with your knees hip width apart. Your hands should be placed directly under your shoulders with your fingers facing forward. Make sure your spine is in neutral position without sagging or arching. Raise your right hip, extending your leg straight out behind you until it is parallel to the floor. Then raise the opposite arm out in front of you until it is parallel to the floor, without tilting your shoulders. You want your core to stay as still as possible and to keep both shoulders parallel to the floor. Gently lower your limbs back to the starting position on all fours and swap sides. Perform this exercise slowly so that you keep your balance.

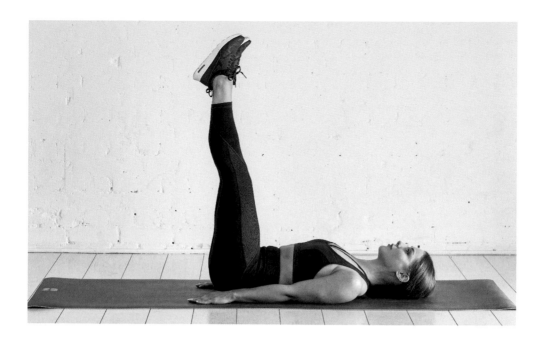

# straight leg raise

- Lie on your back on the floor and place your hands palms down beside your hips. Keep your legs straight and lift them at 90 degrees to the floor. Obviously the higher you bring your legs the more your abs will work, but you don't want to lift your lower back off the ground.

- Lower your legs down towards the floor, but avoid touching it. Hold, then return your legs to the 90 degree angle.

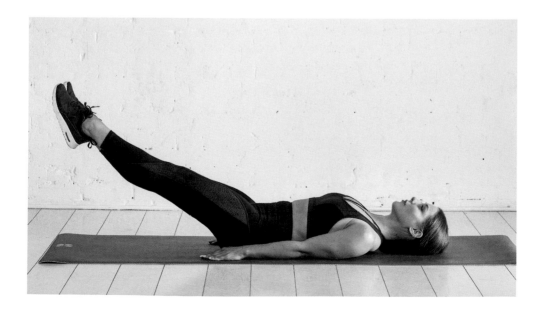

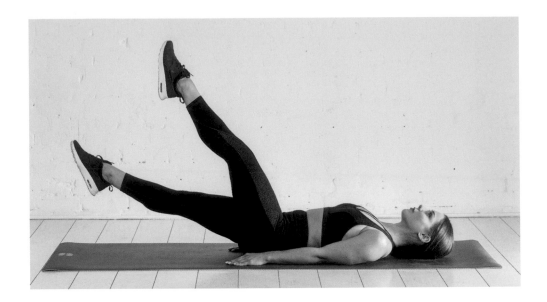

# flutter kicks

- Lie on your back, arms at your sides, legs extended straight and toes pointed away from the body. Raise one leg up to around a 90 degree angle, then as you lower that leg to the start position, raise the other leg, so the legs cross one another. Repeat the movement, making sure you don't allow your feet to rest on the floor, until the rep range is complete.

# scissor kicks

- Instead of kicking up and down, cross your legs over and under one another. Raise both legs up to about 45 degrees off the floor, then (using accuracy so you don't clash feet in the middle) cross one foot over and under the other foot from side to side in a repetitive motion. The larger the range of motion, the more your abs will be working.

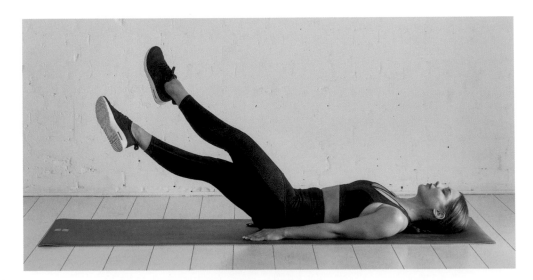

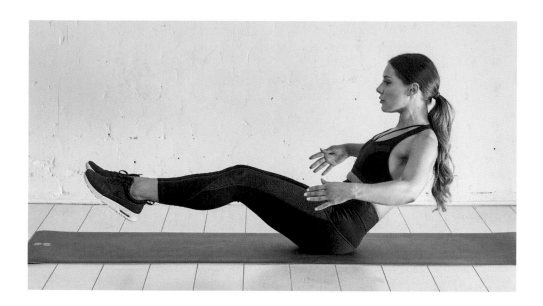

# crunchy frog

I LOVE crunchy frogs – Ryan and I always do them in unison and see how low we can get.

- Sit on the floor in a reclined position, balancing on your bum so that your feet are positioned together and lifted, hovering off the floor. In order to get your feet off the floor you will need to bend your knees and rock back slightly. You might take a bit of time to find your balance. Drive your bent knees towards your chest, and as you do so, take your arms out in front of you and reach them round so that your hands meet in the middle behind your knees. Return to the start position by inhaling, retracting your arms to either side and leaning back as low to the ground as you can but without touching. Repeat.

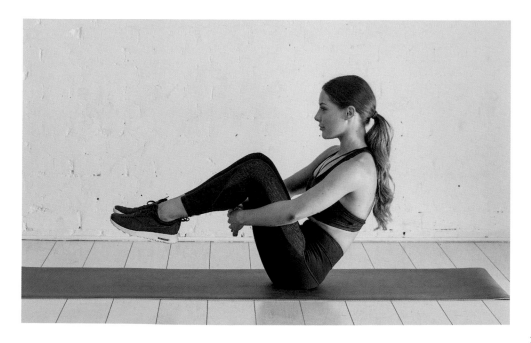

# abs

## crunch

This is probably THE original abs exercise so it's a good one to perfect. Here is a crunch with elevated legs. If you're finding it tough, rest your feet flat on the ground.

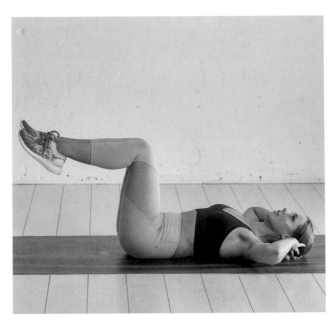

- Lie on your back with your knees bent up at around a 90 degree angle. Put your hands behind your head with your elbows out to the side. Tilt your chin in slightly towards your chest, so that it is tucked in, in order to minimise stress on your neck. Pull your body up towards your knees whilst pulling your abdominals in. Your head, neck and shoulders should lift off the floor.

- People often go the whole way up using momentum to bring them to the top, but I prefer to do a quarter crunch, lifting the top of my back off the floor and then retracting down with a softer landing. Make sure you lower yourself down slowly to avoid hurting yourself.

- Remember that you are pulling your body up using your core and not using your arms to yank your head and neck. Exhale as you sit up, inhale as you come down.

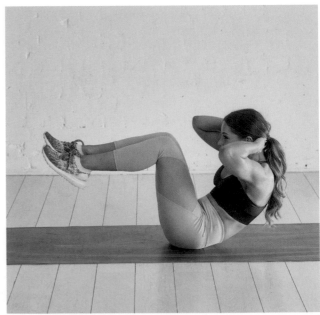

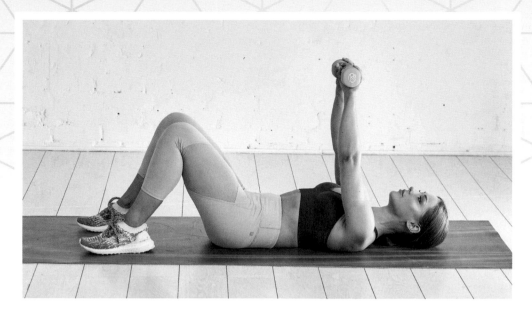

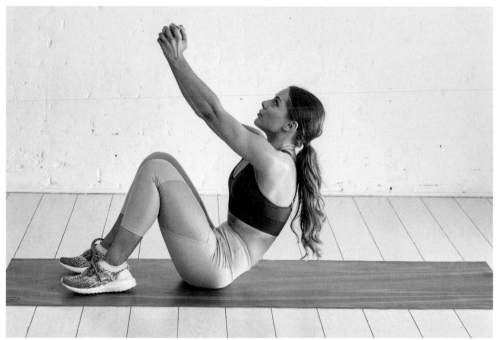

# weighted crunch

I actually prefer doing a weighted crunch to a regular crunch because I like having my hands in front of me driving forwards in an upward motion; it ensures I'm using my abs to lift me and not my back or neck.

- Lie on your back with your knees bent and feet rested on the ground. Hold your arms straight up above your body, holding your weighted object in the middle. Drive the weight upwards (in a crunch) towards the ceiling keeping your arms straight.

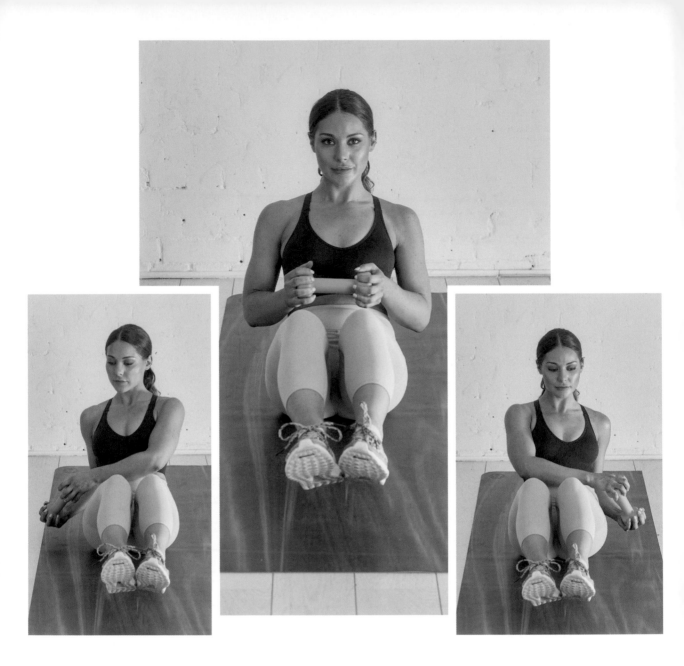

# russian twist

Try starting without a weight to perfect your form, then add a 2kg weight (see above). As you gain strength you can increase the weight.

- Balance on your bum in a comfortable position where your legs are bent and off the ground. This is a similar starting position as a crunchy frog (see 231). Join your hands together in front of your chest and then tap your hands towards the ground on either side of your body, starting with the left then alternating to the right side of your body. You can do this with or without a weight.

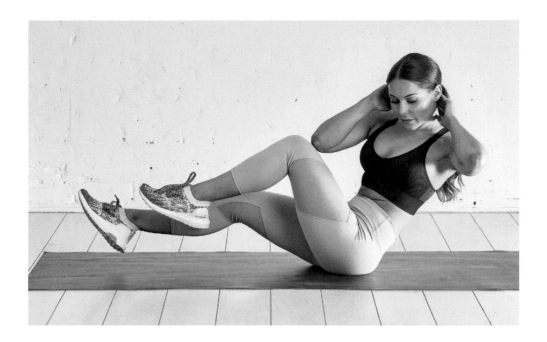

# bicycle crunch

When trying to complete sets it can be easy to speed up without realising, if you slow it down you will reap more benefits because it will test your abs.

*   Get into a crunch starting position (see 232). Reach your opposite elbow across your body to the opposite knee. Your knee and elbow should meet in the middle of your body so both limbs are doing some movement. Move back into the starting position and rotate to the other side.

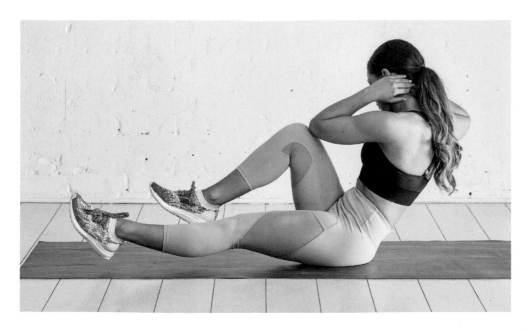

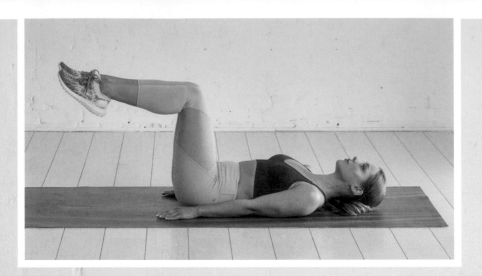

# toe taps

I've learnt that no gym move should be undermined and the power of doing something 'right' can be incredibly effective, no matter how tame it appears – toe taps are a good example of this.

- Lie flat on your back with your arms either side of your body. Bend your knees up to a 90 degree angle, keeping your back flat on the ground (this is called table top position).

- Slowly extend one foot to the ground, tapping the floor with your toes whilst still keeping your back flat to the ground. Then bring that leg back up to table top position and do the same with the other leg. You only want to tap the ground with your toes, not fully rest the foot on the ground.

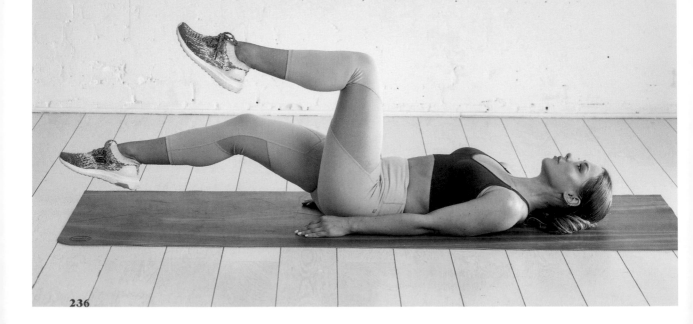

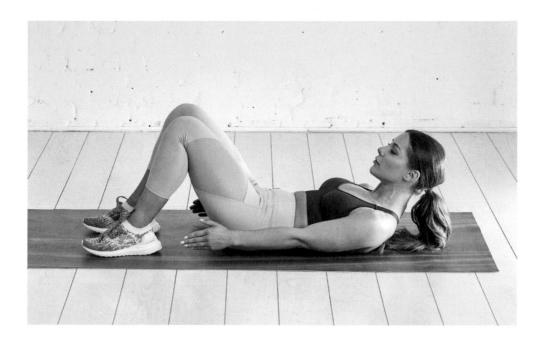

# heel touch

In my ab routine I love when it comes to this exercise because I can catch my breath and have a slight rest. It is a good one for beginners.

- Lie with your back flat to the ground. Lift your neck and shoulders off the ground. Tap your left hand to your left heel. Then tap your right hand to your right heel. Continue alternating. You should feel the burn up the sides of your torso (the obliques).

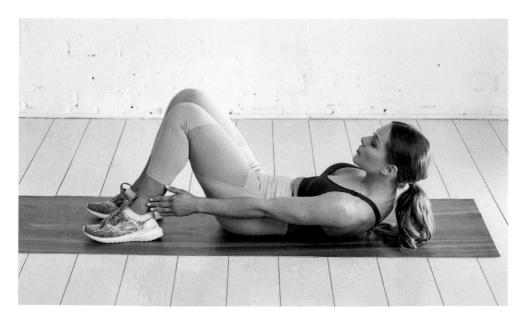

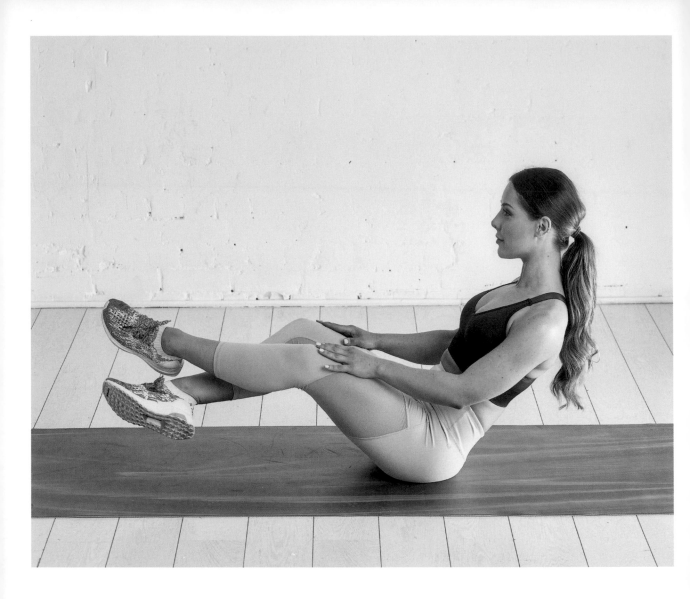

# seated scissor cross

The seated position of this exercise forces you to work harder in order to try to maintain a balanced position.

- Find a comfortable position on your bum with your feet touching the floor, knees bent, next to each other. Then tilt your torso back and try to hover your legs off the ground until you find your balance. Place your hands gently on the top of your thighs. Whilst it might be tempting to hold your legs up by tucking your hands under your thighs, you must avoid this. Then criss cross your feet over and under one another, moving them horizontally.

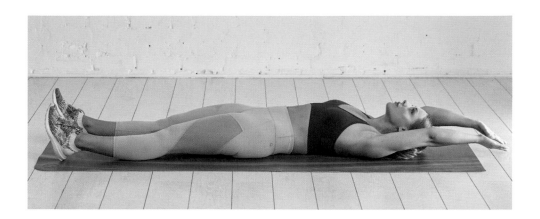

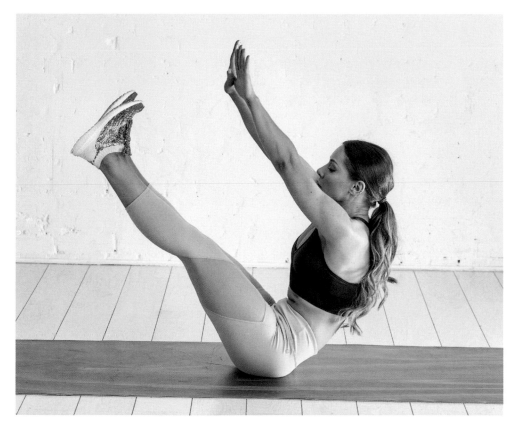

# jackknife

- Lie on your back with your legs and arms outstretched. Keeping them straight, draw your legs and arms up towards each other. You are aiming to raise your legs up to a 45 degree angle and to reach your hands up to touch your toes. Lower slowly, keeping your arms and legs off the floor, repeat until the rep range is complete.

# high intensity

## skipping

Whilst skipping might not be considered the coolest of exercises, it has a whole host of benefits, making it more than worthwhile. I think it is one of the best forms of cardio that can be done at home and without expensive equipment. You can carry a skipping rope in your handbag and you can do it whenever, wherever.

Skipping gives a full-body workout. It also helps with coordination, balance and agility.

- Buy a good-quality skipping rope and adjust it to your size. Hold the handles in each hand by your sides. Keep your shoulders back, chest pushed forward and the weight on the balls of your feet. Then flick the rope forwards by rotating your wrists until you find a consistent motion. Jump, letting the rope pass under your feet.

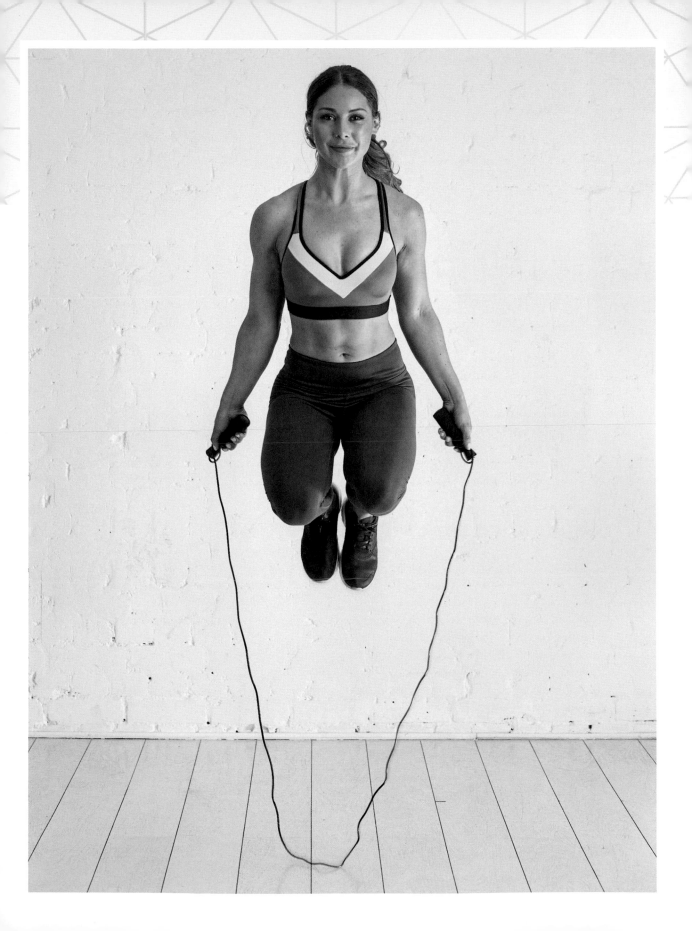

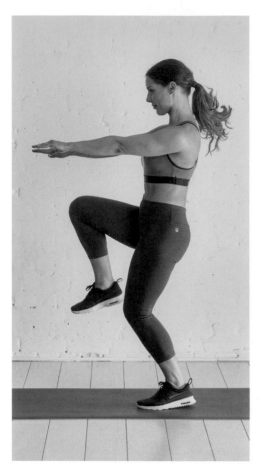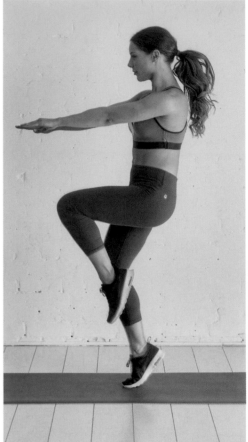

# high-knee running

This cardio move combines lifting your knees as high as possible whilst sprinting as fast as you can. For that reason it is an excellent way to warm-up. This exercise generates a lot of power and burns a lot of energy which is why I recommend doing it for short bursts at any given time. I rarely have the stamina to do it for longer than 30 seconds at maximum capacity. It is an effective way of building strength in your hip flexors and quads, making it a good one to practise if you want to improve your general running ability. Depending on your preference you can either perform the exercise by raising your arms in order to tap your knees as close to your hands as possible or you can use your arms to drive upward in a traditional sprinting pose with your arms either side of your body. I demonstrate the former.

- Begin in a standing position with your arms outstretched in front of you. Raise and lower one knee at a time, reaching hip height. Alternate legs, going as fast and high as you can. You can use your hands to set a target for how high you want to go so that your knees tap them.

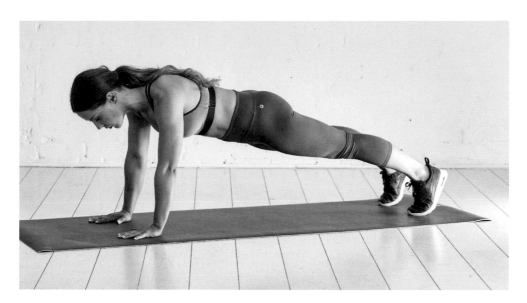

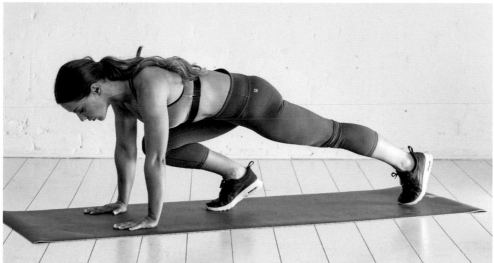

# mountain climbers

This compound exercise provides a great full body workout. It really reminds me of my best friend Binky because whenever we work out together she takes this one VERY seriously and moves like lightening, but making SO much noise.

- Get into a push-up (high plank) position with your arms extended straight and your legs behind you (see page 214). This is your starting position. Then quickly bring one knee towards the back of the same side elbow. In a fast motion, switch legs and do the same with the other leg. As you continue alternating legs the movement should become more explosive.

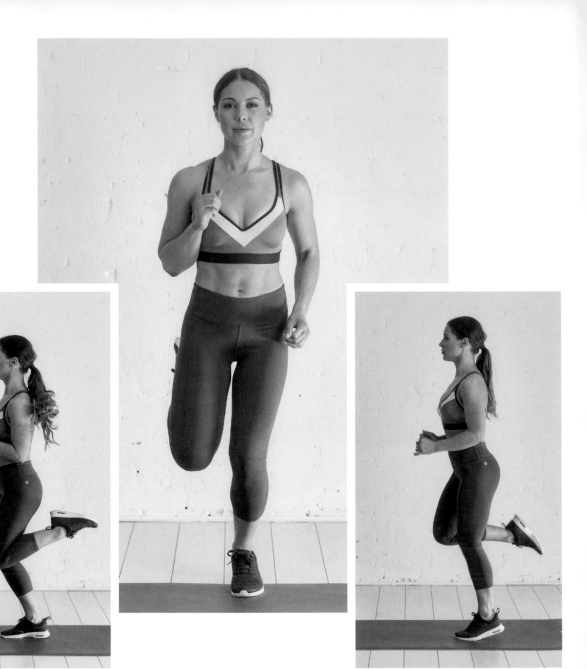

# heel flicks

This exercise is very simple and is a common drill used in football to increase agility and speed.

- Jog on the spot, with your hands behind your back, flicking your heels to kick your bum. Your upper leg should be perpendicular to the floor. The aim is to be as light and quick as possible. This practice is good for encouraging proper running technique, but unlike running can be done in small spaces.

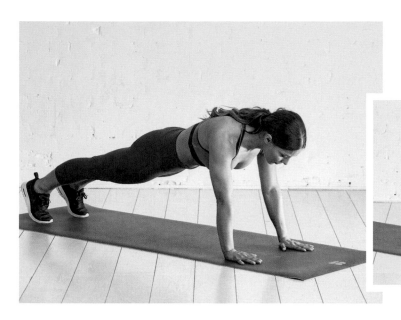

## burpees

Everyone hates burpees and for good reason – they are challenging. But I have decided to include them because they are an effective cardiovascular exercise and train virtually every muscle in your body.

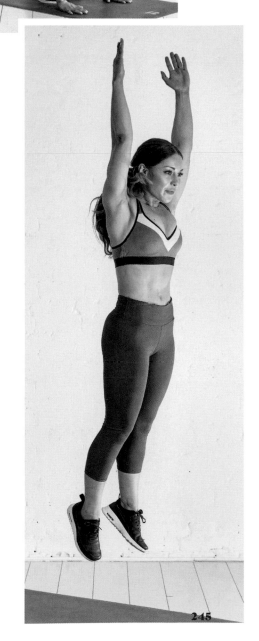

- Stand with your feet shoulder width apart. Jump your feet back into a high plank position.

- Jump your feet in-between your hands whilst bending your knees underneath your hips.

- Explode into a vertical jump, raising your arms in the air. Repeat the movement.

- Speed and power are key for these. However, if you are new to burpees then you can make this exercise easier by moving through the moves at a slower pace, i.e. stepping back into a press-up position as opposed to jumping.

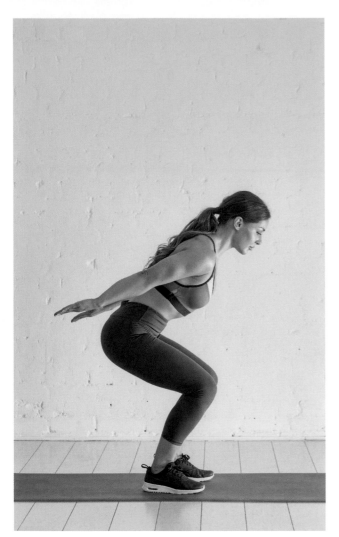
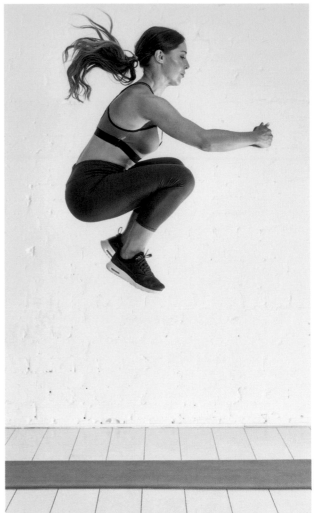

# tuck jump

Tuck jumps are a plyometric exercise, which literally means, 'jump training'. In plyometrics your muscles should exert maximum force during short blasts in order to increase power. Practise these to master them with control.

*   From standing, move into a quarter squat position with your arms stretched out behind your back. Your hips should be back and you should be leaning forwards whilst maintaining a flat back. Immediately explode up, driving your knees up and into your chest. As you do so, bring your arms forwards so your hands meet in the middle, and try to bring your knees as high as your hands.

*   Land on the middle part of your foot and bend your knees when doing so. This will minimise the stress on your knee joints.

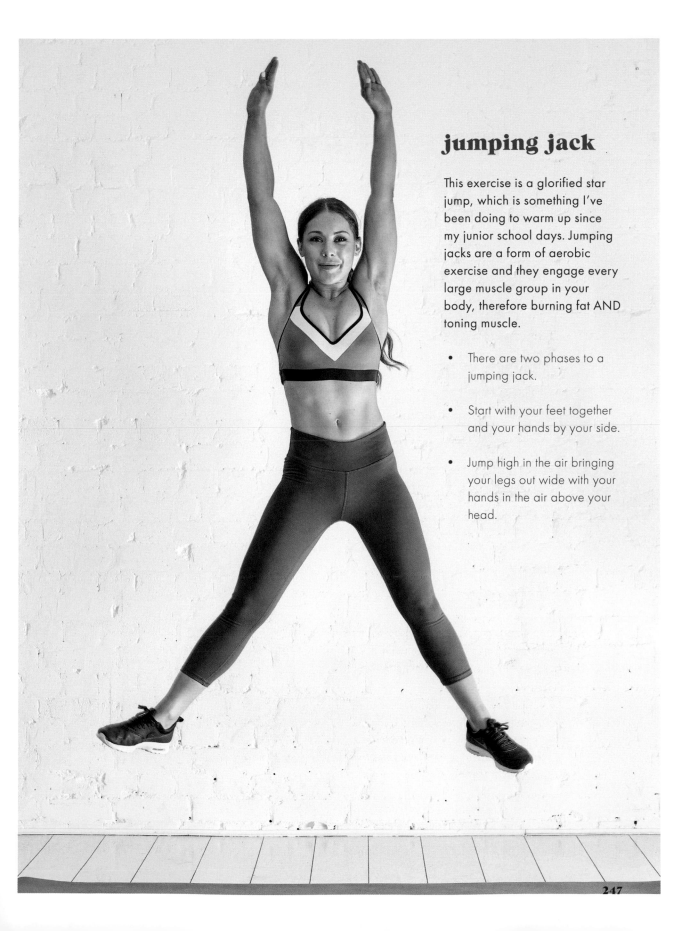

# jumping jack

This exercise is a glorified star jump, which is something I've been doing to warm up since my junior school days. Jumping jacks are a form of aerobic exercise and they engage every large muscle group in your body, therefore burning fat AND toning muscle.

- There are two phases to a jumping jack.

- Start with your feet together and your hands by your side.

- Jump high in the air bringing your legs out wide with your hands in the air above your head.

# cool down

Aim to do 5 minutes of stretching after your workout. This means holding each stretch for 20 seconds in total. Light walking to cool down is a great way to lower your heart rate slowly and safely. If you are in a gym then go for a low intensity walk on the treadmill or if you are at home walk around the room for 5 minutes. This will allow your body to recover and can prevent dizziness.

After your workout IS a good time to do some static stretching, when your muscles are warm. Stretching will minimise pain and muscle fatigue, increase flexibility, blood circulation, and ease tension.

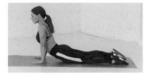

**1. The Cobra Stretch** This yoga pose strengthens the spine, whilst stretching out the chest and abdominals.

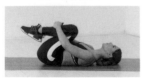

**2. Lower back stretch** Lying on your back, take a few deep breaths and pull both your knees into your chest. Rock back and forward and side to side.

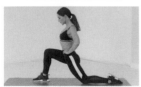

**3. Lunging hip flexor stretch** This stretch is important because your hip muscles play a crucial role in the mobility of the lower extremities.

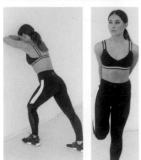

**4. Quad stretch** Stand on your left foot and grab your right foot with your right hand pulling it back behind you. Tuck your pelvis in so that your back isn't curved.

**5. Standing calf stretch** Stand facing a wall a few feet away and bring one foot forward with a slight bend in the knee. Lean towards the wall and rest both arms against it. As you lean forward you should feel a stretch in your calf. Keep your back leg straight and heel down.

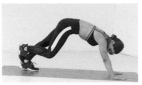

6. **Single leg downward dog** Start in a regular downward dog position and lift one foot off the ground, resting it behind the opposite leg.

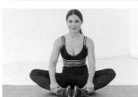

7. **Butterfly stretch** Sitting tall on the floor, place the soles of your feet together so your knees are bent out to the sides. Hold onto your ankles and press your knees down towards the floor. This stretch is good for your hips, thighs and glutes.

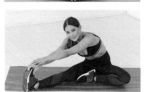

8. **Hurdler hamstring stretch** Sit on the floor with one leg straight out to the side. Bend the other leg in so that the sole of your foot is in contact with your inner thigh. Lift your arms above your head and reach forward towards the foot of the straight leg.

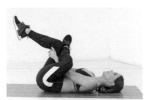

9. **Glute stretch** Lie on your back and lift your left hip and leg and cross it over your right leg so that it is resting just above the knee. Keep your back and shoulder flat on the ground and lift your right leg using your hands. The further you pull your right leg into your body the stronger the stretch.

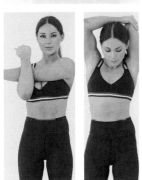

10. **Tricep stretch** Extend your arms overhead. Bend your left elbow and reach your left hand towards the middle of your back. Reach the right hand overhead and bend to hold the left elbow, gently pulling down on it.

11. **Shoulder stretch** Stand tall with your feet shoulder width apart. Place your left arm across your chest so that it is parallel to the ground. Bend your right arm up and use the forearm to pull the left arm closer to your chest. You should feel a gentle stretch in your left shoulder.

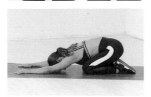

12. **Child's pose** This stretches the hips and thighs as well as relaxing the back muscles and the muscles at the front of your body. Breathe out whilst lowering your hips to your heels. Reach your forehead toward the floor. Stretch your arms out above your head with your palms on the floor. Breathe slow and deep.

# index